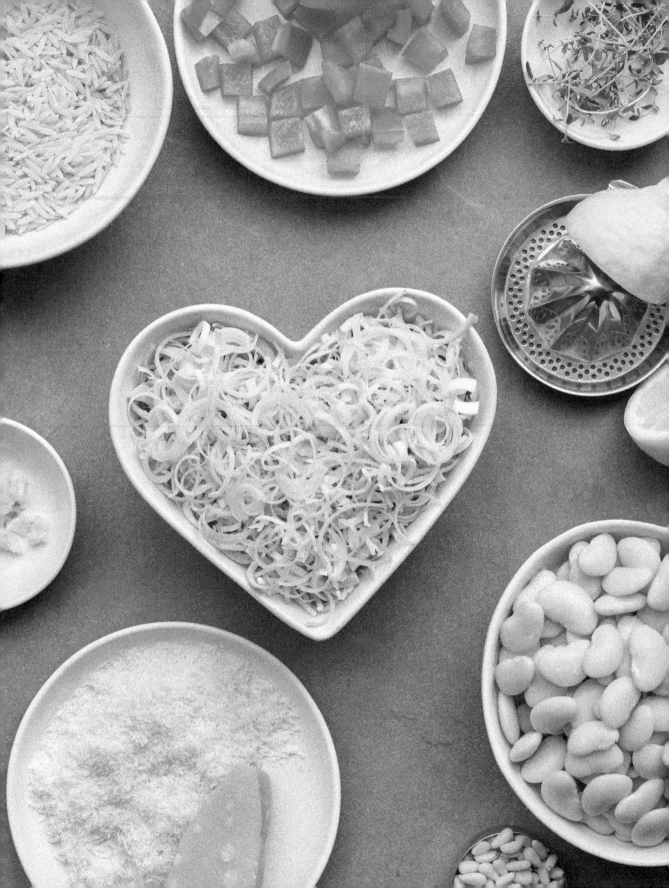

30-MINUTE
HEART HEALTHY
COOKBOOK

Delicious Recipes for Easy,
Low-Sodium Meals

BY CHERYL STRACHAN, RD

PHOTOGRAPHY
DARREN MUIR

ROCKRIDGE
PRESS

To my generous mother, Lynda, who helps without hesitation when needed; Kayla, for the late-night chats; Nicole, for the early-morning snuggles; and Blair, who tackles one pile of dishes after another with a wink and a smile.

First Rockridge Press trade paperback edition 2019

Rockridge Press and the Rockridge Press logo are trademarks or registered trademarks of Callisto Media Inc. and/or its affiliates in the United States and other countries and may not be used without written permission.

For general information on our other products and services, please contact our Customer Care Department within the United States at (866) 744-2665, or outside the United States at (510) 253-0500.

Paperback ISBN: 978-1-64152-632-6 | ebook ISBN: 978-1-64152-633-3

Interior and Cover Designer: Eric Pratt
Art Producer: Sue Bischofberger
Editor: Clara Song Lee
Production Manager: Riley Hoffman
Production Editor: Melissa Edeburn
Photography © 2019 Darren Muir
Author photo © Janet Pliszka

10 9 8 7 6 5 4 3 2 1

CONTENTS

INTRODUCTION

People with heart concerns have been my focus since I became a dietitian 14 years ago and began practicing in a cardiac rehabilitation program. I facilitate nutrition classes and counsel cardiac patients and their families after heart health scares. These days, I also have a private practice focused on prevention and helping people who have a family history of heart disease or who want to address risk factors like high cholesterol and blood pressure.

If you or a family member recently had a cardiac event or have been struggling with a heart disease risk factor, you might be feeling worried, scared, or even angry right now. People ask: How could it have been prevented? Could I have eaten differently? Exercised more? Worked less? Lost a few pounds?

Regardless of the answers, it's never helpful to blame yourself. Numerous factors contribute to heart disease, including many over which we have little control. Family history, race, and age are well-known factors, but other determinants of health are becoming more widely recognized, including childhood experiences, education, social status, and income. Even the so-called modifiable risk factors are really only somewhat changeable. For example, often our bodies don't maintain weight loss; our communities and jobs aren't always set up to promote movement or healthy eating.

The good news is that after a heart-related diagnosis, most people survive—and even thrive—for many years. There are no guarantees, but you *can* influence your destiny. Staying active, managing stress, attending cardiac rehabilitation programs, and eating well have all been shown to reduce the incidence of future heart problems. These practices can also boost your energy and add joy to your life.

Over the years I've had the pleasure of working with local cardiac support groups and rehab program volunteers, getting to know many people who continue to live happily for 25 years or more after a cardiac event. Most are relatively healthy eaters, but they're not perfect, and you don't need to be either.

I believe in walking the talk, so heart-healthy living—in particular, eating—is a priority in my life. For 11 years now, I've also been a working mother, figuring out how to feed a busy family without sacrificing nutrition or, just as importantly, our enjoyment of food.

Many of my clients struggle with similar challenges. Who has the time to cook everything from scratch? Temptations surround us, from doughnuts in the break room to chocolate in the pantry. Every package in the grocery store seems to be loaded with sodium or sugar. Advice on what to eat, much of it conflicting, comes at you from every direction.

This book helps you take control of the critical nutritional driver of heart health with simple, satisfying recipes designed to help you follow three similar, plant-based, heart-healthy eating patterns: DASH, Mediterranean, and vegetarian/vegan.

The recipes have been designed for speed and efficiency, so you can make them even when you're short on time or energy. Within 30 minutes you can be enjoying a meal made with easy-to-find, affordable ingredients. Many of the recipes in this book call for just five ingredients, and most require no more than ten.

Are you ready to feed yourself and your family easy, delicious meals that will provide energy and promote heart health? Let's get started.

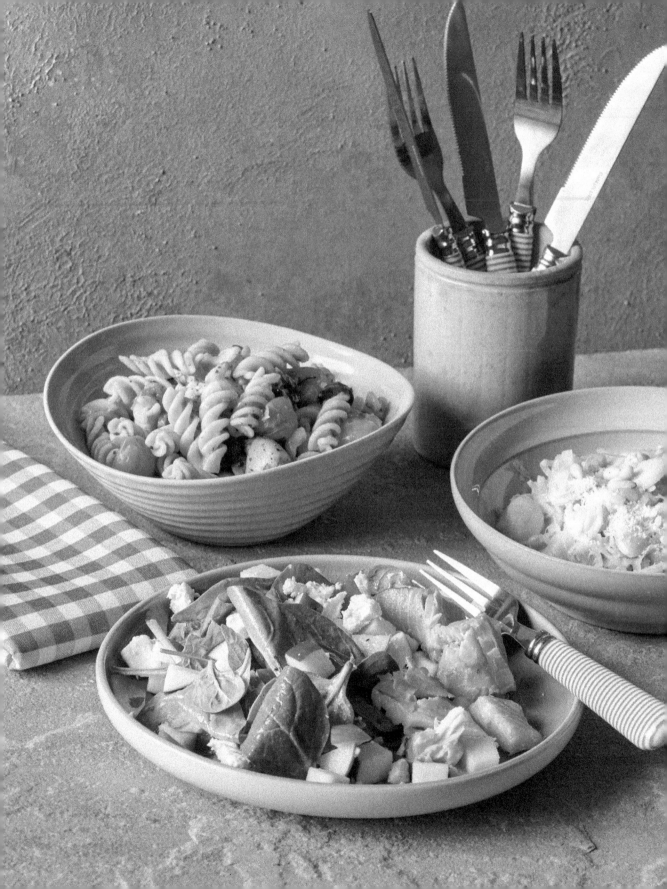

CHAPTER ONE

HEART-HEALTHY EATING

If you want some clarity around how to eat to support heart health, start here. I'll summarize the state of the evidence and be frank about what's still unclear. Then we'll talk about fundamental tools and skills that can make you a heart-healthy home chef in no time.

When we talk about the heart, we often really mean the cardiovascular system—the blood vessels that supply our bodies with life-giving blood and oxygen. Over the years they can become narrowed and hardened, which may eventually lead to a blockage, like a major pileup on the highway.

A blockage in one of the vessels, or arteries, delivering blood to the heart results in a heart attack. In the brain, it's known as a stroke. In the legs, it's called peripheral arterial disease.

Although the catchall term "heart disease" can also refer to other problems, like a faulty valve or infection in the heart, cardiac nutrition guidelines generally focus on the health of those all-important arteries.

CARING FOR YOUR HEART THROUGH FOOD

Whether you've had a blocked artery or are concerned about your risk for one, think of this as an opportunity to prioritize *you* for a change. You can't change every risk factor for heart disease, but most people have some control over their food choices. And your eating habits can make a difference.

- In the Lyon Diet Heart Study, for example, 605 heart attack survivors were randomly assigned to follow either a **MEDITERRANEAN** eating pattern or a prudent Western diet. Over the next four years, 14 people in the Mediterranean group had another heart attack or died from cardiac causes, compared to 44 in the control group. Other cardiovascular problems were also reduced in the Mediterranean group.

- A 2013 meta-analysis (study combining the results from several studies) found that people whose diet most closely matched the Dietary Approaches to Stop Hypertension (**DASH**) eating pattern were 20 percent less likely to develop cardiovascular diseases than those whose diet least closely matched the DASH pattern.

- A 2012 meta-analysis found that **VEGETARIANS** were 29 percent less likely to die from ischemic heart disease (heart problems caused by narrowed heart arteries) than nonvegetarians.

WHY CAN'T THE EXPERTS AGREE?

You've likely noticed that nutrition advice seems ever-changing—yes or no on meat, eggs, butter, coconut oil, carbs, etc.—depending on who's dispensing it.

Why does this happen? First, people are drawn to controversy, so ideas that go against conventional wisdom dominate the headlines and sell more books. The same goes for celebrities, who often follow and promote extreme diets. Fans are drawn to their physical beauty, which usually has more to do with genetics and socioeconomic advantage than what diet they follow.

Second, food packages and advertisements communicate subtle nutrition information, which can be misleading. The food industry also funds research, which influences what gets studied and published.

Third, cardiac nutrition research is complicated and imperfect. Consider the complexity of heart disease, which develops over decades with countless contributing factors.

Three meals a day add up to more than a thousand meals a year, each made of potentially dozens of ingredients and hundreds of nutrients. In addition, food is intimately tied to other aspects of our lives, which can affect heart disease. Is cheese heart-healthy? The answer will be different if you're in the habit of eating it on take-out pizza on your couch or with fruit on a hike with friends.

Science has various approaches for untangling all of this, few of which give definitive answers. The many nutrition studies are like pieces of a puzzle. Sometimes the results are consistent and the picture is fairly clear. Every year we add a few more pieces to the puzzle and our understanding evolves.

WHAT TO DO?

The good news is that the *fundamentals* of eating for heart health are reasonably well understood and agreed upon. So what can you do when you hear something that contradicts what you think?

CONSIDER THE SOURCE. Is the information coming from a nutrition expert? (Unfortunately, most doctors aren't nutrition experts.) Has the source considered all of the evidence, not just one study? Is the source's goal to grow a large television or online audience, which takes drama and novelty, or is it to truly educate? Are they selling something?

WHEN IN DOUBT, GO WITH MODERATION. When the evidence isn't clear, it's often because the food, in reasonable amounts, doesn't have a major effect one way or the other. You can use this strategy for eggs, butter, alcohol, even bacon.

FACTOR IN YOUR PREFERENCES. What do you enjoy? What foods leave you feeling energized? What foods align with your values and lifestyle? These considerations matter as much as the more direct health effects.

TRUST YOURSELF AND DO WHAT WORKS FOR YOUR BODY. You know yourself best.

WHAT YOUR HEART LOVES

A heart-healthy eating pattern is one that doesn't stress you out.

To reduce your risk for future heart problems, fuel yourself primarily with a variety of minimally processed plant foods, including plenty of vegetables, fruit, whole grains, nuts, seeds, and legumes/beans. Fish, dairy, and lean meat can help, too, as long as they fit into your overall dietary preferences.

Focus on incorporating these cardioprotective foods, and you'll find yourself naturally easing up on refined grains, added sugars, red and processed meat, and sodium. Moderation of alcohol is warranted, as well, if you drink at all.

WHY, HOW, WHERE, and **WHEN** you eat matter as much as **WHAT** you eat. Habits like cooking, sharing meals with others, honoring cultural traditions, and taking a few minutes to relax and enjoy your food can contribute to heart health more than kale and lentils. Practice eating away from the TV or other distractions so you truly experience the satisfaction of eating and notice when you start to fill up.

Your body also needs **SLEEP** and **RELAXATION** for heart health and to support healthy eating. Studies have shown that people intentionally deprived of sleep eat hundreds of extra calories. When you're tired, the last thing you may want to do is cook. And although eating to soothe difficult emotions isn't necessarily a problem, if you do it so often that it affects your well-being, learning other strategies may help. Nutrition is important, but it's not so critical that it should prevent you from enjoying food with loved ones or become a source of worry or angst. A heart-healthy eating pattern is one that doesn't stress you out.

Depending on your health situation, other approaches may also be useful. I'll briefly outline them here. But remember, the information in this book is general in nature. If you have any cardiac risk factors that aren't well controlled, or other conditions like diabetes, chronic kidney disease, or digestive problems, consider working individually with a registered dietitian nutritionist (RDN) or other healthcare professional.

HIGH CHOLESTEROL

If high LDL (bad) cholesterol is a concern, choosing foods with more **UNSATURATED FATS** and less **SATURATED FATS** may help. As a basic rule, that means getting more fat from plant foods like olive oil, nuts, seeds, and avocados, and less from animal foods like butter and prime rib. The exceptions are fish, an animal with mostly healthy fats that should be included in your diet, and coconut and palm oils, which are plant-based but full of mostly cholesterol-raising saturated fats and should therefore be left out.

SOLUBLE FIBER, found in foods like oats, pears, flax, and legumes, can help, too. You'll find plenty of these foods in the recipes in this book.

Some people's blood cholesterol goes down when they reduce their intake of **CHOLESTEROL**-rich foods like eggs, meat, and shrimp, but for most it has little effect. **SOY PROTEIN** helps, but it takes quite a bit to make a difference. Dietary efforts can lower your cholesterol by about 20 percent, but cholesterol levels are largely inherited, so don't be surprised if your doctor encourages you to take medication for it, despite your best efforts.

HIGH TRIGLYCERIDES

If high triglycerides are a problem for you, again, eating foods rich in **UNSATURATED FATS** can help. Cut back on nutrient-poor, carbohydrate-rich foods, like sweetened drinks, juice, white rice, and white flour–based baked goods. It may help to cut back on or stop drinking alcohol. Enjoy more fish, nuts, seeds, and whole grains.

HIGH BLOOD PRESSURE

High blood pressure? Reducing **SODIUM** is the first thing people think of, but instead of the salt shaker, focus your attention on restaurant and packaged foods. Adding ¼ teaspoon of salt to a meal for four adds about 150 milligrams (mg) of sodium each, whereas restaurant meals can easily top 2,000 mg, with some as high as 4,000 mg.

The American Heart Association recommends no more than 2,300 mg of sodium a day, and ideally no more than 1,500 mg for most adults, especially those with high blood pressure. (For the rest of us, it's about prevention.) The World Health Organization and Hypertension Canada suggest 2,000 mg or less.

Worrying about your exact sodium intake isn't necessary for most people. Just cook at home more, eat out less, and limit your intake of packaged foods with more than 15 percent sodium listed on the label. Most of the recipes in this book contain less than 500 mg of sodium per serving, some well below, to help you get there. It takes time for your palate to adjust to lower-sodium food, so be patient and cut back gradually if that helps.

The other effective strategy for lowering blood pressure is the **DASH** eating pattern; see more about that on page 10. Finally, cutting back on alcohol may also help if you frequently have more than a couple of drinks a day.

DIABETES AND PREDIABETES

With type 2 diabetes and prediabetes, people's first instinct is to limit sugar, but that's just one aspect of blood sugar–friendly eating. It also helps to spread out your meals in general, and all **CARBOHYDRATES** in particular, over the course of the day, eating at least three meals as well as a small snack or two if needed.

Other aspects of heart-healthy eating are appropriate for people with diabetes, as well, including eating fruit and limiting fruit juice. Studies show that even people with diabetes who eat more than three servings of fruit a day live longer.

Guidelines for managing type 1 diabetes are beyond the scope of this book. Work with your healthcare team, including a registered dietitian nutritionist.

WEIGHT LOSS

Take any advice to lose weight with a grain of salt. We have much less control over body size and shape than conventional wisdom suggests. Some people can lose weight with diet and exercise changes, but few keep it off for longer than a year or two. (Medication and surgery can be more effective, but these methods aren't available to or appropriate for everyone.) Interestingly, although studies show that weight loss can improve heart disease risk factors, which change relatively quickly, we have no evidence that losing weight helps people live longer or avoid further cardiac problems in the long run.

You may be thinking, "What's the harm in trying?" First, frustration with weight loss can make people abandon exercise and healthy eating, both of which have been shown to benefit heart health even when weight doesn't change. Second, repeated cycles of weight loss and gain are associated with increased rates of heart disease, as well as emotional and disordered eating. The prevalence of binge eating disorder, for example, is higher in people with a history of dieting for weight loss. And ironically, one of the best predictors of weight gain is dieting.

If **BETTER HEALTH** is your goal, instead of defining success by pounds lost, focus on what you *can* control: exercising, getting enough sleep, relaxing, taking your medications, and of course, eating healthy.

MEDICATION-FOOD INTERACTIONS

Check with your pharmacist to confirm any food interactions with the medications you're taking. Here are some common interactions:

- If you take **WARFARIN**, you may have been advised to keep your intake of vitamin K consistent. The recipes in this book list the amount of vitamin K to help you familiarize yourself with the relative levels. Your vitamin K intake doesn't have to be precisely constant, but you should avoid sudden, significant changes.

- Certain cardiac medications come with advice to limit **POTASSIUM**. If that's a concern, you can refer to the potassium values under each recipe in this book. (If your potassium is high due to poor kidney function, a renal diet cookbook may be more helpful.)

- Finally, some cardiac-lowering medications may interact with **GRAPEFRUIT**, grapefruit juice, and other fruits, so you won't find those ingredients in this book.

POPULAR HEART-HEALTHY EATING PATTERNS

Three dietary patterns (Mediterranean, DASH, and vegetarian/vegan) have been shown to improve cardiac outcomes, and they have many more similarities than differences. Here are the core components to aim for:

BASE YOUR MEALS ON VEGETABLES, FRUITS, OR BOTH. This isn't a new idea, but it's still a challenge for most people. Ideally, vegetables and fruit should make up about half of every meal and snack; if that's not realistic for you, start with a little and build from there.

EAT LEGUMES, NUTS, AND SEEDS ON MOST DAYS. Legumes include lentils, chickpeas, dried peas, and beans. Tofu, made from soybeans, counts, too. Experiment with nut and seed butters, from peanut butter to tahini. These plant-based-protein foods have consistently been tied to improvements in cardiac risk factors and outcomes.

CHOOSE MOSTLY WHOLE GRAINS. All three dietary approaches include a moderate intake of grains, mostly whole. Bread products are a start, but challenge yourself to try intact grains like oats, quinoa, and barley, which can be cooked without salt and which are generally easier on your blood sugar.

MAKE EXTRA-VIRGIN OLIVE OIL YOUR FIRST CHOICE. Extra-virgin olive oil is a feature of the Mediterranean diet in particular, but it makes sense no matter which approach you use, unless you're cooking at very high temperatures for a long time, as when searing meat, stir-frying, or roasting in the oven at 400°F or higher. Heart-healthy oils that withstand high temperatures better include canola, sunflower, grapeseed, and avocado.

AIM FOR AT LEAST TWO SERVINGS A WEEK OF FISH. Fatty fish, including salmon, trout, and sardines, are especially beneficial.

These three well-studied dietary patterns are all variations on the themes I've just listed. Beyond these general principles, there's more flexibility than you might think.

MEDITERRANEAN

The Mediterranean diet is really a general eating pattern practiced in different ways around the Mediterranean region. In addition to the core components just outlined, it's characterized by wine with meals—although the relative importance of this is unclear. The small potential cardiac benefits of wine should be weighed against the considerable risks of excess. Even moderate amounts of alcohol are associated with an increase in breast cancer risk, for example.

Otherwise, Mediterranean diets are typically higher in fat than the other two, but most of it comes from sources like fish, olive oil, and nuts. Red meat is consumed infrequently, and poultry, eggs, and dairy make weekly rather than daily appearances. The Mediterranean lifestyle also involves slowing down to enjoy meals with others and getting plenty of physical activity.

DASH

The Dietary Approaches to Stop Hypertension (DASH) pattern of eating was first popularized after two well-designed studies looked at its effect on blood pressure in the late 1990s. Since then, it has been studied extensively relative to other aspects of cardiac health, with consistently positive results.

The diet is quite high in vegetables and fruit—8 to 10 servings a day for typical adults—as well as whole grains, nuts, seeds, legumes, and mostly low-fat milk products. Meat, fish, chicken, eggs, and vegetable oils are included, but in smaller amounts than is typical in the standard American diet.

Since the original studies, researchers have varied the DASH pattern and seen similarly positive results. One study looked at higher-fat milk products. One reduced carbohydrates slightly and replaced them with either more plant-based protein or healthy fats.

The bottom line is that, as long as you include the core components, you can vary the specifics as per your preferences.

VEGETARIAN/VEGAN

There is a great deal of interest in vegetarian and vegan diets, thanks to passionate researchers, dramatic documentaries, and concerns about environmental sustainability and animal welfare. Vegetarians do not eat any meat, including chicken and fish. Vegans go a step further and don't eat any food of animal origin, from dairy products to eggs and even honey.

Evidence tying these approaches to cardiac outcomes is limited but promising. Cardiologist Dean Ornish showed a reversal of atherosclerosis (arterial disease characterized by deposits of fatty materials) in people randomly assigned to a very low-fat, nearly vegan diet, along with smoking cessation, stress management, and moderate exercise. Atherosclerosis in the control group got worse.

Although the degree of reversal was small, the clinical effect was significant, showing that people in the control group were twice as likely to experience a cardiac event during five years of follow-up. However, because this was a small study and participants did more than just change their diet, we can't say for sure that a low-fat vegan diet is the only way to reverse atherosclerosis. If a vegan diet appeals to you, consider consulting a registered dietitian nutritionist to ensure you meet all of your nutrient needs.

WHAT ABOUT LOW-CARBOHYDRATE EATING PATTERNS?

Various low-carbohydrate diets have surged in popularity over the years, from Atkins to paleo, South Beach to the currently popular ketogenic diet. Even the rise in gluten-free eating was driven by a low-carb undercurrent, in addition to legitimate gluten intolerance among a small percentage of people.

These diets are popular because they typically result in rapid, although usually temporary, weight loss and the improvement in cardiac risk factors—such as type 2 diabetes, blood pressure, and cholesterol—that goes with it. Unfortunately, as noted earlier, the weight lost usually returns.

Given that we have few studies examining these approaches beyond two years, and none showing reductions in cardiac events or improved mortality, I don't typically recommend them. If, however, such an approach appeals to you, and you think you can realistically eat that way long-term, it is possible to take a heart-healthy approach to it. Load up on nonstarchy vegetables, nuts, seeds, avocado, fish, and lean meat. Consider working with an RDN to ensure you meet your nutritional needs.

EATING PATTERNS: THE BOTTOM LINE

Which approach you take matters less than what these eating patterns have in common. A 2013 study that examined the eating habits of more than four thousand heart attack survivors found that moving to any type of heart-healthier diet was associated with 30 percent lower all-cause mortality and 40 percent lower cardiovascular mortality.

Components of the diet tied to better outcomes in that study were vegetables, fruits, nuts, legumes, whole grains, unsaturated fats, and a reduction in red and processed meats, sugar-sweetened beverages, alcohol, trans fat, and sodium.

FIVE PRINCIPLES OF HEART-HEALTHY EATING

1. **FOCUS ON SATISFACTION FIRST.** This might seem counterintuitive, but if you're eating in a way you don't truly enjoy, it won't last for long. Take time to explore and experiment with new foods and try different recipes. If you can find food that truly gives you pleasure, you may well continue eating this way for the rest of your life, and that's the goal.

2. **NOURISH YOUR BODY.** Healthy eating is not about restriction. Instead, think about fueling your body and focusing on cardio-protective foods. A nutritious, balanced meal or snack at least every four to five hours can help keep your energy up and your appetite in check. If you can avoid getting too hungry, you may find it easier to avoid overeating later.

3. **LET GO OF FOOD GUILT AND RELAX.** Your diet doesn't have to be perfect. In fact, aiming for that is usually counterproductive. Labeling certain foods as "bad" or "off-limits" can cause a *"restrict and binge"* cycle when we inevitably slip. Instead, give yourself unconditional permission to eat all foods, including the ones you think of as "bad." You may soon find they lose their power over you.

4. **DON'T MEASURE YOUR SUCCESS BY WEIGHT LOST.** As we've discussed, dieting for weight loss sets you up for failure. The pursuit of better health is about what you do, not what you weigh.

5. **AIM FOR *YOUR* SWEET SPOT.** What I call the sweet spot is simply what works *for you*—food that you enjoy, that supports your health, and that works in other ways that matter to you, like convenience or sustainability. Getting to your sweet spot can take time, but it will be worth it. You deserve to not only survive, but truly live. And good food is part of a full life.

HEALTHY PORTIONS
FOR A HEALTHY HEART

Chronically eating more than your body needs can contribute to weight gain and increase your chances of developing prediabetes and type 2 diabetes, both of which are heart disease risk factors.

The best guide to how much you should eat is you. Our appetites ebb and flow, and we are all born with the ability to self-regulate.

However, in our harried, supersized, diet-centric, waste-averse, food-saturated environment, it's easy to lose touch with feelings of hunger and fullness. A bit of structure and guidance can be helpful.

The illustrated portion sizes that follow are guidelines, not hard and fast rules. When in doubt, honor your hunger.

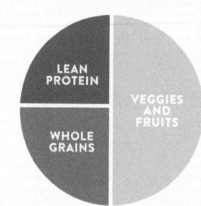

This heart-healthy, balanced plate is a simple approach to meal planning. The idea is that about half of each meal should be vegetables and fruit. Adding one or two sources of protein can help you feel full and provide valuable nutrients. The rest of the meal, about a quarter of what you eat, can be grains, mostly whole, or starchy vegetables like potatoes.

FOODS AND THE ROLES THEY PLAY

In their quest for better heart health, people often have questions about specific foods: Is avocado okay? What about eggs?

The table on page 16 addresses these questions. **STARS** are foods that have been consistently shown to help improve heart disease outcomes. Base your meals around them. Complement them with the **SUPPORTING CAST** foods, which are fine to eat in moderation if you like. Or skip them. Either way, eating too much from the supporting cast column can crowd out the cardioprotective stars.

CAMEO APPEARANCE foods are chosen for perfectly good reasons other than health: holiday cookies to celebrate tradition, a deli sandwich as you're dashing to catch a plane, or macaroni and cheese just because. How much you eat is up to you. Some people think in terms of the 80/20 principle (80 percent of the time you're eating with health as the priority, 20 percent is more about pleasure or convenience); some prefer to be more or less conservative. Some weeks you'll be on vacation; some weeks you'll be settling back into your routine.

Your mind-set can make a difference. Remember that you're *allowed* to eat those cameo foods. *You* decide, factoring in your preferences and personal circumstances. You might *choose* to eat them less often. Or not. No one should judge you for your food choices, even after a health scare.

Don't think of any foods as good or bad. It's more about balance—how much and how often. A slice of bacon crumbled in a colorful salad is not the same as three slices with eggs and buttered white toast every morning. Your overall eating pattern matters more than particular foods or nutrients.

FOODS FOR HEART-HEALTHY EATING

STARS (the show revolves around these)	SUPPORTING CAST (play a role but shouldn't steal the show)	CAMEOS (small but enjoyable appearances, if you're a fan)
• Extra-virgin olive, canola, sunflower, grapeseed, and avocado oils • Homemade salad dressing with these oils	• Soft spreads and margarine with no hydrogenated oils (check the ingredients list) • Store-bought salad dressing • Mayonnaise	• Butter • Coconut oil • Palm oil
• Still and low-sodium carbonated water • Unsweetened herbal teas	• Unsweetened caffeinated tea and coffee • Alcohol in moderation	• Soda • Sweetened iced tea, lemonade • Flavored coffees • Other sweetened drinks
• Unsweetened milk (the lowest fat level you enjoy) and yogurt, especially plain Greek yogurt • Plain kefir (the lowest fat level you enjoy)	• Flavored Greek yogurt • Cheese • Fortified plant beverages with about 12 grams of sugar or less per cup	• Chocolate and other sweetened milks (the lowest fat level you enjoy) • Processed cheese • Regular flavored yogurt • Yogurt drinks and flavored kefir (the lowest fat level you enjoy)
• Vegetables: fresh, frozen, or canned (without added sauce, salt, or seasonings) • Fruit: fresh or frozen • Avocados	• Vegetables in sauce or canned with salt • Vegetable juices without added salt • Starchy vegetables like potatoes, sweet potatoes, and corn • Fruit smoothies: Aim for about 1 cup of fruit per serving and include foods with protein, like milk or peanut butter.	• French fries, potato chips, and other fried vegetables • Vegetable juice with salt added • Fruit juice, even if it's unsweetened • Dried fruit • Prepared spaghetti sauce

STARS (the show revolves around these)	SUPPORTING CAST (play a role but shouldn't steal the show)	CAMEOS (small but enjoyable appearances, if you're a fan)
• Intact whole grains, such as farro, bulgur, oats, brown or wild rice, quinoa, and barley • Sprouted-grain bread • Whole-wheat pasta and couscous • Whole-grain crackers such as "Hint of Salt" (low-sodium) Triscuits and rye crispbread (such as Wasa)	• Whole-grain bread and bread products (look for a whole grain at the start of the ingredient list) • Whole-grain, high-fiber cereals like Cheerios and All-Bran Buds • Pasta cooked al dente • Instant oatmeal, granola	• White rice • White bread and bread products (enriched wheat flour is the first ingredient) • Refined-grain crackers, baked chips • Refined-grain cold cereals, including Corn Flakes, Special K, Rice Krispies • Gluten-free grain products with rice starch or potato starch as the first ingredient • Sweetened grain products like muffins, scones, cookies, and cakes
• Dried Legumes, including dried peas, beans, lentils, edamame (soybeans), and tofu • Canned legumes with no salt added, rinsed and drained • Nuts and seeds, including nut and seed butters, ideally natural • Fish, especially salmon, trout, sardines, and other fatty fish	• Legumes canned with salt, hummus • Canned fish, shellfish, and lower-sodium fish sticks • Skinless chicken and turkey, light or dark meat • Lean beef, pork, and lamb cuts (such as round or loin) • Organ meats • Wild game • Eggs • Vegan meat substitutes	• Reduced-fat peanut butter • Battered, fried fish • Poultry skin • Chicken wings and fingers • Duck and goose • Sausages, bacon, lunch meat, and other processed meats • Ribs, rib eye, and other fatty beef, pork, and lamb cuts
• Vinegars, lemon and lime juice • Lemon or lime zest • Cooking wine • Hot peppers • Dried and fresh herbs • Spices • Salt-free seasoning mixes	• Reduced-sodium soy sauce and tamari • Hot sauce • Table, kosher, and sea salt, in small amounts • Reduced-sodium broth or soup base • Dark chocolate and unsweetened cocoa	• Restaurant and takeout food • Sweets • Milk chocolate

HEALTHY FOOD FAST

Whether eating with heart health in mind is new to you or a practiced habit, I want to help you enjoy it. I've designed the recipes in this book with satisfaction, ease, and affordability in mind. Whichever of the heart-healthy eating approaches you're drawn to, you'll find a variety of ways to experiment and build your repertoire. My goal is that you'll find the recipes satisfying and energizing enough that you'll look forward to eating them, regardless of health considerations.

TEN TIPS FOR QUICK AND EASY MEALS

Can you really get a delicious, heart-healthy meal on the table in half an hour? Absolutely! The recipes in this book will get you there—all of them take 30 minutes or less. But the following tips (and a little practice) can help you be more efficient with any recipe:

1. Before you start, take a minute to read all the way through the recipe and gather the ingredients.

2. Preheat the oven or start a pot of water boiling if needed, so they'll be ready when you are.

3. Start with whatever meal component takes the longest to cook, such as barley or brown rice.

4. If time is short, aim to include just a vegetable, a protein-rich food, and a starch—whole-grain or vegetable. You can add more for flavor and variety, but the shorter your ingredient list, the sooner you'll be eating.

5. Experiment with cooking at higher temperatures. Roasting at 400° to 450°F or even judiciously using the broiler can save time and give food a nice, crispy exterior.

6. Leave the skin on produce such as apples and potatoes to eliminate an unnecessary step and retain heart-healthy fiber, vitamins, and minerals. You may even find that you prefer the heartier texture.

7. If possible, prepare everything—protein, vegetables, and grains—in one dish. You can add broccoli or frozen shrimp to pasta while it's cooking, if you get the timing right. Salads, stews, chilis, and soups can all be quick, heart-healthy, one-pot meals.

8. Roasting or baking? Skip the scrubbing by lining your pans with parchment paper. It's generally compostable, nonstick, and oven-safe to 420°F. At higher temperatures, use aluminum foil.

9. Save even more time on busy weeknights by preparing some components on weekends or whenever you have a bit more time and energy. Cook brown rice or other grains, and freeze it in small containers. Cook chicken, baked potatoes, or vegetables like butternut squash, which take time but require little hands-on effort.

10. Double whatever you're cooking. If you won't eat it in two or three days, freeze the leftovers in small containers so you can defrost faster. Take a minute to label them so they don't get lost in the freezer.

ON-THE-GO SNACKS

Heart health is about much more than what you eat. Relaxing, connecting with others, and spending time outdoors supports your health and makes life worth living. Instead of waiting until you can plan the perfect menu, be spontaneous and invite a friend for a picnic in the park or dinner on the deck. The following is a list of snack ideas that you can pack and eat while you are out and about with friends or family.

RINSE-AND-GO VEGETABLES: baby cucumbers, cherry tomatoes, fresh peas, mini bell peppers, broccoli or cauliflower florets

PROTEIN TO GO: spiced or caramelized or salted roasted nuts, Dark Chocolate and Cherry Trail Mix (page 161), Happy Heart Energy Bites (page 162), canned sardines, tuna packed in oil*, cheese, rotisserie chicken, hard-boiled eggs (look in the deli section)

WHOLE GRAINS: fresh whole-grain bread, whole-wheat rolls, whole-grain crackers

SPREADS: cashew dip, roasted red pepper dip, hummus, baba ghanoush, olive tapenade, peanut butter

NO-PREP FRUIT: grapes, oranges, berries, fresh-cut fruit from the market

DRINKS: ice water, flavored carbonated water, unsweetened coffee or tea

DESSERT: dark chocolate, Banana-Oatmeal Cookies (page 169)

*Canned fish like sardines and tuna are usually salted, but they're also full of omega-3 fats and protein. If you like them, balance them with lower-sodium foods like fruit and vegetables.

THE CONVENIENT COOK'S KITCHEN

If cooking hasn't been a priority in your life until now, this all might feel a bit overwhelming. Fear not! Here is a brief guide to essential kitchen tools, pantry staples, simple meal planning, and shopping with heart health in mind. You've got this.

BASIC KITCHEN EQUIPMENT

You don't need cupboards full of pots and pans and fancy kitchen equipment to make the recipes in this book. I've pared it down to the following 15 basics:

1. **KNIVES.** You will need an 8- to 10-inch chef's knife for chopping and slicing and a 3- to 4-inch paring knife for small, fine cuts. If yours aren't sharp, have them sharpened professionally, buy a small handheld sharpener, or replace them.

2. **CUTTING BOARDS.** Plastic and wood are both fine, but reserve one for fresh fruit and vegetables and another for raw meat and poultry. (A third one for onions and garlic helps keep those strong flavors to themselves.)

3. **POTS AND PANS.** Key pieces include a large, deep sauté pan or skillet with a lid, a large pot, and a rimmed baking sheet.

4. **COLANDER.** You'll need this to rinse beans and vegetables and strain pasta. Start with a big one that stands up on its own, and add a handheld fine-mesh strainer for rinsing smaller items like quinoa or lentils, if needed.

5. **MEASURING CUPS AND SPOONS.** Metal is more expensive but sturdier and longer-lasting. Look for long, narrow measuring spoons that fit into spice jars.

6. **BLENDER OR FOOD PROCESSOR.** Either of these appliances will easily purée smoothies, soup, dips, and sauces. Some food processors can also slice or grate, saving time on preparing vegetables and cheese.

7. **MIXING BOWLS.** Glass is microwave-safe, but stainless steel is lighter; pick whatever works for you. (If you buy pretty ones, they can double as serving bowls.) Lids are a bonus.

8. **INSTANT-READ FOOD THERMOMETER.** This gadget is a must for getting big pieces of lean meat, poultry, or fish to a safe internal temperature without overcooking.

9. **MICROWAVE OVEN.** A microwave will reheat, thaw, and even cook food more quickly and with less nutrient loss than other cooking methods. Some people are suspicious about the effect of microwaves on health, but there is no evidence to suggest that foods prepared in the microwave are harmful.

10. **BOX GRATER.** A box grater is more stable and easier to handle than a handheld grater, and you can use it for shredding cheese and vegetables like carrots, and for shaving the intensely flavored outer skin of citrus fruits like lemon.

11. **BASTING BRUSH.** You'll use this tool for brushing oil on baking dishes and sauce on food.

12. **CAN OPENER.** Whether handheld or electric, this is a must-have for convenience foods like canned tomatoes, beans, and fish.

13. **WOODEN SPOONS AND WIRE WHISK.** Both of these tools will do the trick for mixing.

14. **SPATULA AND TONGS.** You'll need one or the other for turning hot food.

15. **VEGETABLE PEELER.** Depending on the model, you'll use this tool for peeling vegetables and then shaving them or even cutting them into long, thin strips, making interesting textures for salads.

PANTRY ESSENTIALS

These basic, affordable items are used over and over in the recipes in this book. High-quality frozen, canned, and dried items are excellent ingredients—they are generally inexpensive, healthy, and convenient.

FRESH

- Apples and oranges are a good source of soluble fiber and a portable snack

- Extra-firm tofu, to boost the protein in any meal (see Crispy Tofu, page 186)

- Sun-dried tomatoes packed in oil (look for 60 mg of sodium per tablespoon or less) make a quick pasta dish with chicken and vegetables

- Pesto, to drizzle over fish or replace pizza sauce (look for one with less than 400 mg of sodium per ¼-cup serving, or make your own Walnut Pesto, page 181)

- Reduced-sodium soy sauce or tamari, for a quick boost of savory taste (look for one with 600 mg sodium per tablespoon or less, and use sparingly)

- Hard block of flavorful cheese, such as Parmesan; freshly grate it over anything from roasted vegetables to a tossed salad

- Onions, garlic, and ginger; these aromatic vegetables are cooked at the start of many recipes to impart flavor, and they are especially important when you're using less salt

- Lemon and lime juice for tart, tangy flavor, or finely grated zest for a sweeter, more intense citrus flavor

FROZEN

Many fruits and vegetables are flash-frozen right after being picked at the height of freshness, so they're nutritious, often have no added salt or sugar, and work well in many cooked dishes.

- Corn, chopped onions and peppers, mixed stir-fry vegetables

- Fruit, such as berries, mango, and ripe bananas you've peeled and frozen yourself

- Nuts and seeds stay fresh much longer in the freezer than at room temperature

CANNED

Canned foods may have more salt than fresh, but many no-salt-added alternatives are widely available, so look for them. You can make a quick, healthy meal out of canned food in a pinch.

- No-salt-added tomatoes

- Beans

- Salmon and tuna

- Reduced-sodium chicken or vegetable broth in a can or box; or use a reduced-sodium base like Better Than Bouillon

- Herbs and spices, for seasoning food with less salt

- Whole grains such as rice, barley, pasta, and quinoa

- Fruit, including cranberries, apricots, and plums for snacking or for adding sweetness to foods like oats and salads; dried fruit is very sugar-dense, so think of it as a sweet condiment used sparingly rather than a replacement for fresh or frozen fruit

GROCERY STORE GUIDE: HOW TO SHOP

Shopping after a new diagnosis of heart disease can be stressful. You may feel as if you have to examine every package under a microscope. But don't worry; before long you'll have discovered new favorites, and shopping will become routine again.

Start with a meal plan. There's no need to plan every bite, but selecting even two or three main meals to cook can help you be more efficient. Check your fridge, freezer, and pantry first, so you don't double up on things you already have. If your budget is tight, scan the weekly supermarket flyers and incorporate sale foods into your plan.

Then, use your plan to make a shopping list, adding staples and snacks. If you create one on the computer, you won't have to write the same items week after week. Organize it by section, and you'll zip through the store in no time. Visit my website (sweetspotnutrition.ca) for free meal planning and shopping list forms that you can download and customize for yourself.

Be aware of powerful merchandising and marketing tactics aimed at luring you into buying more than you planned. How food is displayed, sampled, packaged, and priced can influence what ends up in your cart. Billions of dollars are spent every year, from commercials to product placements in movies and magazines. You may not think they affect you, but there's a reason food companies spend that money.

One strategy is offering shoppers many choices. An average super-market in 2017 carried more than thirty thousand items. There are sixteen varieties of Cheerios on Walmart.com today! More options usually lead to more purchases.

So, what can you do?

- **SHOP AFTER EATING.** You've heard it before, and it's true. If necessary, stash some nuts or granola bars in the car to help you stick to your list.

- **CONSIDER SHOPPING ONLINE.** Any extra cost may be offset by fewer impulse buys and time saved.

- If you want to cut down on sweets and salty snacks, consider **NOT BUYING THEM REGULARLY.** You can indulge when you like, but not having them in the house makes it intentional instead of mindless eating.

- **CONSIDER A STORE WITH FEWER OPTIONS,** like Trader Joe's or Costco. Their buyers have made the choice for each category, so if you like their products, you can reduce the "overwhelm factor."

In some ways, healthy eating can cost more, but there are ways to save. Don't pay a premium for ill-defined benefits like *natural* or *artisan*. In my opinion, pricier organic and non-genetically modified (non-GMO) food isn't necessary for good health. Gluten-free packaged foods usually cost more and are needed only if you have a gluten-related health condition such as celiac disease.

Compare unit prices. Bigger packages are usually a better deal, but we tend to eat more from them, potentially negating any savings. And don't buy more than you'll realistically use. Wasted food is wasted money.

Produce is generally more affordable (and nutritious) when it's in season, so keep an eye on prices. Prep vegetables for snacks right after you get home, and store them at eye level in the refrigerator so they're more likely to be eaten than composted.

READING LABELS

When reading the "Nutrition Facts" table on food packages, look at the following:

- **SERVING SIZE.** If you're judging whether a food has a little or a lot of a nutrient, remember to consider how much you actually eat, which may be different from the serving size on the label.

- **CALORIE** is a loaded word, but it's simply a measure of food energy. Make sure you get enough to fuel yourself, rather than thinking of calories as the enemy.

  The easiest way to interpret most of the numbers is to focus on the % Daily Value, which tells you how much of a nutrient the food contains relative to the needs of a typical adult. Five to ten percent or less is considered low, whereas 15 to 20 percent or more is on the high side.

- **SATURATED FAT** raises LDL cholesterol. **TRANS FATS** do, too, and have other harmful effects on vascular health. They're combined to give one % Daily Value. Look for a low number here.

- **SODIUM** is a good one to check, to help prevent and manage high blood pressure. Again, look for a low number.

- **DIETARY FIBER** includes the parts of plant foods your body can't digest or absorb. It goes in one end and out the other, helping to lower LDL cholesterol, stabilize blood sugars, and support gut health. Look for a higher number.

continued

- **TOTAL SUGARS.** Excess sugar intake is associated with higher rates of heart disease, stroke, type 2 diabetes, and high cholesterol. Labels in the United States now also include **ADDED SUGARS,** sweeteners added by the manufacturer, which health guidelines recommend most adults limit to about 50g.

- **PROTEIN.** There is no % Daily Value for protein; aim for at least 20g to 30g for a meal and 8g to 10g for a snack to help you feel full and slow down age-related muscle loss.

HEALTHY STORE-BOUGHT SHORTCUTS

If saving time in the kitchen is important to you, it may be worth paying a bit more for certain convenience foods that sacrifice little in the way of health and taste:

- Meat or chicken cut into strips make for quick stir-frying or sautéing; frozen chicken breasts pounded thin also cook quickly.

- Prewashed greens, such as spinach, baby kale, and others, can be added to a number of dishes to boost nutrition.

- Bagged salad is ready to dump into a salad bowl; then, consider using just half the dressing or tossing with extra-virgin olive oil and vinegar.

- Precut fruit and vegetables are great for snacks or stir-fries; use within a day or two.

- Frozen vegetables, including broccoli, spinach, kale, and even butternut squash, will save you lots of prep time—new products seem to appear every week, so check your supermarket.

- Herb, garlic, and ginger stir-in pastes let you add flavor to dishes in seconds.

- Fully or partially cooked brown rice and other whole grains are available plain so you can season them yourself (the flavored products are usually high in sodium).

- Rotisserie chicken can be the beginning of many quick meals; although most have added salt, the sodium is usually lower than deli meat, and you'll avoid nitrates and nitrites.

- Frozen meals with whole grains, vegetables, beans, fish, and chicken beat takeout on those hectic evenings when from-scratch cooking just isn't going to happen. Look for sodium levels close to 600 mg or less. Generally healthier brands include Luvo, Trader Joe's, Healthy Choice, Amy's, and Evol.

ABOUT THE RECIPES

My goal is to help you feel more confident and relaxed about cooking, so most recipes in this cookbook have just 10 ingredients or fewer, and all can be on the table within 30 minutes. Some have as few as five ingredients, can be made in just one pot, or both, and are labeled accordingly.

I designed the recipes around cardioprotective foods like vegetables, fruit, legumes, whole grains, nuts, healthy fats, and fish. Most use minimally processed, shelf-stable, convenient, affordable foods you'll find at your neighborhood grocery store.

Recipes labeled "Portable" are things that you can pack up and eat on the go as is, no reheating necessary. Recipes tagged with the DASH and Mediterranean labels include the components in those dietary patterns that most people typically don't get enough of, like vegetables, whole grains, and nuts and seeds. The Mediterranean diet recipes aren't all flavored like traditional Mediterranean dishes, but they will help you practice this pattern of eating.

You'll find nutrition information, as well, to give you confidence that nutrients like sodium and saturated fat fall within cardiac guidelines. Most meet the following parameters:

CALORIES: about 500 per serving for entrées

SODIUM: 500mg or less per serving for entrées and even less for sides and snacks

SATURATED FAT: 5g or less per serving

ADDED SUGAR: 8g or less per serving

I did the nutrition analysis using ESHA Research's Food Processor software. The numbers include all optional ingredients; if two options are given, I've done my calculations using the first.

I wish you well. Cook, eat, enjoy, and go on living your life!

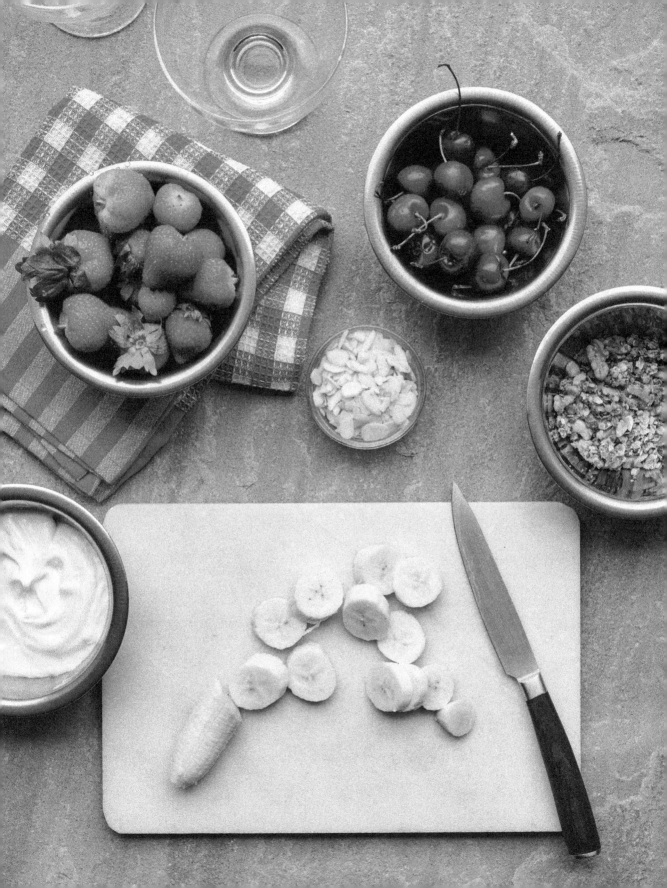

STRAWBERRY BREAKFAST SUNDAE 34

CHAPTER TWO

BREAKFASTS AND SMOOTHIES

STRAWBERRY BREAKFAST SUNDAE

DASH • MEDITERRANEAN • VEGETARIAN • 5-INGREDIENT • NO-COOK • PORTABLE

This sundae is perfect for those mornings when you're short on time but still want a nutritious and delicious breakfast. Because flavored yogurt has about 3 teaspoons of added sugar per cup, this recipe uses plain yogurt and sweetens the dish with banana, strawberries, and granola. If you want it even sweeter, add a drizzle of honey or pure maple syrup. The sundae looks beautiful served in a wine glass—or, for a quick weekday breakfast, spoon it all into a container and off you go.

Serves 2

Hands-on time: 5 min

Total time: 5 min

1 cup plain 2% Greek yogurt, divided

1 banana, sliced, divided

½ cup Omega-3 Skillet Granola (page 41) or store-bought low-sugar granola, divided

¼ cup slivered almonds, divided

1 cup strawberries, divided

1. Divide the yogurt between two bowls.
2. Top each with half of the sliced banana, granola, almonds, and strawberries.

SUBSTITUTION TIP: This recipe works well topped with any berries, whether fresh or frozen and thawed. Look for frozen dark cherries, too.

INGREDIENT TIP: Greek yogurt with 2% fat is creamier than nonfat, and 5% is even better. This small amount of saturated fat is unlikely to make a difference to heart health, so choose the one you like best.

PER SERVING: Calories: 415; Total Fat: 22g; Saturated Fat: 4g; Cholesterol: 18mg; Sodium: 91mg; Carbohydrates: 33g; Fiber: 7g; Added Sugars: 0g; Protein: 20g; Potassium: 711mg; Vitamin K: 5mcg

CHOCOLATE POWER SMOOTHIE

DASH • MEDITERRANEAN • VEGAN • NO-COOK • PORTABLE

Frozen blueberries and spinach give you a morning nutrition boost. Substitute whatever kind of milk you prefer. If you go with cow's milk, you may need a teaspoon or two of honey to sweeten it. If you go with almond milk or another plant beverage, which are very low in protein, double the hemp seeds.

Serves 2 (1½ cups per serving)

Hands-on time: 10 min

Total time: 10 min

1 medium frozen banana

1 cup baby spinach

1 cup frozen blueberries

2 tablespoons unsweetened cocoa powder

2 tablespoons natural peanut butter

1½ cups vanilla soy milk

1 tablespoon hemp seeds

¼ to ½ cup water (optional)

1. If you don't have a very powerful blender, roughly chop the banana.

2. Combine the banana, spinach, blueberries, cocoa powder, peanut butter, soy milk, and hemp seeds in the blender, and purée very well. Add the water, a few tablespoons at a time, if you prefer a thinner consistency.

INGREDIENT TIP: Shelled hemp seeds (sometimes called hemp hearts) have a nutty, earthy taste and are high in protein and heart-healthy fats. Buy them in the natural food aisle of a well-stocked grocery store, or in any health food store.

FLAVOR BOOST: Exchange the peanut butter for a cup of chilled brewed coffee for a mocha delight.

PER SERVING: Calories: 285; Total Fat: 13g; Saturated Fat: 2g; Cholesterol: 0mg; Sodium: 180mg; Carbohydrates: 37g; Fiber: 8g; Added Sugars: 5g; Protein: 12g; Potassium: 812mg; Vitamin K: 89mcg

BLUEBERRY-BANANA SMOOTHIE

DASH • MEDITERRANEAN • VEGETARIAN • NO-COOK • PORTABLE

Frozen mango gives this classic combination a fresh twist, and the Greek yogurt and hemp seeds provide a morning protein boost. Buy whatever fat level you prefer on the yogurt—or leave it out entirely to make this a vegan smoothie. If you still want the extra protein, you can add a bit of vegan protein powder.

Serves 2 (2 cups per serving)

Hands-on time: 10 min

Total time: 10 min

1 banana

1 cup frozen blueberries

½ cup frozen mango chunks

2 cups vanilla soy milk

½ cup plain 2% Greek yogurt

2 tablespoons hemp seeds

Combine the banana, blueberries, mango, soy milk, yogurt, and hemp seeds in a blender, and blend well.

PER SERVING: Calories: 281; Total Fat: 8g; Saturated Fat: 1g; Cholesterol: 3mg; Sodium: 141mg; Carbohydrates: 41g; Fiber: 5g; Added Sugars: 5g; Protein: 17g; Potassium: 814mg; Vitamin K: 19mcg

BANANA KEFIR SMOOTHIE

DASH • VEGETARIAN • 5-INGREDIENT • NO-COOK • PORTABLE

Researchers are just beginning to understand the important role our gut bacteria and other microorganisms play in our metabolic and cardiovascular health. We still have much to learn, but it appears that fermented foods with live, active cultures, such as kombucha, kimchi, and kefir, may be helpful not only for gut health, but also for heart health. The bananas in this smoothie provide sweetness and blood pressure–friendly potassium. This recipe also works with frozen mango chunks or cherries.

Serves 2

Hands-on time: 5 min

Total time: 5 min

1½ cups plain, unsweetened dairy kefir

2 small frozen bananas

2 teaspoons honey (optional)

1. Mix the kefir and bananas in a blender until smooth.

2. Taste, and add honey if needed.

INGREDIENT TIP: Kefir (a fermented milk) is one of the richest food sources of live, active cultures, but flavored dairy kefir is high in sugar and plain kefir tastes too sour for many people. Still, given the protein, calcium, and other nutrients it offers, in addition to the friendly microbes, it's worth experimenting with.

PER SERVING: Calories: 194; Total Fat: 2g; Saturated Fat: 1g; Cholesterol: 10mg; Sodium: 82mg; Carbohydrates: 38g; Fiber: 3g; Added Sugars: 6g; Protein: 9g; Potassium: 695mg; Vitamin K: 1mcg

PEANUT BUTTER AND RASPBERRY TOAST

DASH • MEDITERRANEAN • VEGAN • 5-INGREDIENT • PORTABLE

This quick breakfast can help you get deliciously fueled and on with your day. Pair it with a glass of milk and you'll have more than 20 grams of protein—a nutrient often in short supply at breakfast. Natural peanut butter has the heart-healthiest fats and no sugar or other fillers. Look for oil on top and nothing but peanuts and possibly some other nuts on the ingredients list. Just stir in the oil at room temperature and then store the jar in the fridge. If it gets dry toward the bottom of the jar, stir in a bit of canola or sunflower oil.

Serves 1

Hands-on time: 5 min

Total time: 5 min

1 slice sprouted-grain bread

2 tablespoons natural peanut butter

1 teaspoon hemp seeds (optional)

¼ cup fresh raspberries

1. Toast the bread.

2. Spread the peanut butter on the toast. Sprinkle with hemp seeds (if using). Top with the raspberries.

INGREDIENT TIP: Bread made from sprouted grain has more protein and less impact on blood sugar than whole-wheat bread. It's so hearty that one slice is plenty for most people.

PER SERVING: Calories: 344; Total Fat: 18g; Saturated Fat: 3g; Cholesterol: 0mg; Sodium: 184mg; Carbohydrates: 29g; Fiber: 8g; Added Sugars: 0g; Protein: 13g; Potassium: 186mg; Vitamin K: 2mcg

SALMON AND AVOCADO TOAST

This hearty breakfast can help you get closer to two servings a week of fatty fish. Canned salmon is convenient and relatively affordable, and it usually contains environmentally friendly wild-caught fish. Having a higher-protein breakfast like this one may help you feel full for longer and keep your muscles strong as you age. Pair it with a cup of berries, and you'll be ready to take on the day.

Serves 3

Hands-on time: 15 min

Total time: 15 min

1½ whole-grain bagels, split

1 (7.6-ounce) can sockeye salmon, drained

1 tablespoon extra-virgin olive oil

1 avocado, peeled and pitted

1 tablespoon freshly squeezed lime juice

½ cup chopped fresh tomatoes

¼ cup minced red onion (optional)

Freshly ground black pepper (optional)

1. Toast the bagels.

2. Meanwhile, in a medium bowl, mix the salmon with the olive oil, breaking up the pieces.

3. In a small bowl, mash the avocado with the lime juice.

4. Top each toasted bagel half with some salmon mix. Spread the avocado on top of the salmon, followed by the tomatoes, then onion and pepper (if using).

COOKING TIP: If you have leftover cooked salmon, lucky you! Use that instead. Or try smoked salmon—it's higher in sodium but still a good source of omega-3 fatty acids.

PER SERVING: Calories: 366; Total Fat: 18g; Saturated Fat: 3g; Cholesterol: 47mg; Sodium: 463mg; Carbohydrates: 27g; Fiber: 7g; Added Sugars: 0g; Protein: 27g; Potassium: 659mg; Vitamin K: 15mcg

PEACH-CRANBERRY SUNRISE MUESLI

DASH • MEDITERRANEAN • VEGAN • NO-COOK

Here's a refreshing, cholesterol-friendly start to the day when it's too hot to cook oats. Muesli is like overnight oats for those of us who don't manage to plan breakfast the night before. Substitute nectarines or peaches canned in water or juice if you can't find good fresh peaches, or try it with Blueberry-Chia Jam (page 184). You can boost the protein by adding a spoonful of Greek yogurt, a hard-boiled egg on the side, or even a scoop of protein powder.

Serves 1

Hands-on time: 5 min

Total time: 15 min

⅓ cup vanilla soy milk

3 tablespoons rolled oats

1 tablespoon chia seeds

1 tablespoon buckwheat (optional, see tip)

1 peach

1 tablespoon dried cranberries

1 tablespoon sunflower seeds

1. Mix the soy milk, oats, chia seeds, and buckwheat (if using) in a large bowl. Soak for at least 10 minutes (and as long as overnight).

2. Meanwhile, cut the peach into bite-size pieces.

3. When the oats have softened up, sprinkle with the cranberries, sunflower seeds, and peach chunks.

INGREDIENT TIP: Packages of buckwheat may also be labeled buckwheat groats. Buckwheat is a gluten-free whole grain that adds a crunchy texture; if you can't find it, just use more oats.

LEFTOVERS: Make a larger batch (8 servings) by mixing 1½ cups oats with ½ cup each sunflower seeds, chia, buckwheat, and cranberries. Store in an airtight container in the refrigerator, and spoon out about ½ cup at a time. Soak with ⅓ cup vanilla soy milk, and then top with your choice of fresh fruit when you serve it.

PER SERVING: Calories: 361; Total Fat: 11g; Saturated Fat: 1g; Cholesterol: 0mg; Sodium: 42mg; Carbohydrates: 59g; Fiber: 12g; Added Sugars: 21g; Protein: 13g; Potassium: 669mg; Vitamin K: 6mcg

OMEGA-3 SKILLET GRANOLA

DASH • VEGETARIAN • ONE POT • PORTABLE

This granola is low in sugar compared to what you'll typically find in the supermarket, and it's lovely paired with fruit or yogurt. You can also use it to jazz up plain cereal, like puffed or shredded wheat. Flaxseed and chia seeds are here for their omega-3s; hemp seeds are more notable for their protein. The flax and chia also contribute fiber, particularly cholesterol-lowering soluble fiber. You should be able to find these ingredients at many supermarkets and at all health food stores; if not, substitute whatever you have on hand.

Serves 4 (½ cup per serving)

Hands-on time: 10 min

Total time: 10 min

2 tablespoons Better Butter (page 176) *or* 1 tablespoon canola or sunflower oil plus 1 tablespoon unsalted butter

1 tablespoon honey

¾ cup large-flake rolled oats

⅓ cup roughly chopped walnuts

1 tablespoon chia seeds

1 tablespoon hemp seeds

1 tablespoon ground flaxseed

½ teaspoon ground cinnamon

Pinch salt

1. In a large skillet, melt the Better Butter and honey over medium heat, then continue to cook until bubbly.

2. Stir in the oats, walnuts, chia seeds, hemp seeds, flaxseed, cinnamon, and salt and cook, stirring, until the oats and nuts start to brown, 3 to 4 minutes. If they're browning too fast, turn the heat down to medium-low.

3. Eat the granola right away or let it cool completely, then store in an airtight container for up to 2 weeks in the pantry or 3 months in the freezer.

SUBSTITUTION TIP: For a vegan granola, use extra oil and pure maple syrup instead of the butter and honey.

FLAVOR BOOST: Add a few dried cranberries, raisins, or unsweetened coconut flakes after cooking.

PER SERVING: Calories: 230; Total Fat: 16g; Saturated Fat: 3g; Cholesterol: 8mg; Sodium: 64mg; Carbohydrates: 18g; Fiber: 4g; Added Sugars: 4g; Protein: 5g; Potassium: 157mg; Vitamin K: 3mcg

ALMOST-INSTANT OATMEAL

DASH • MEDITERRANEAN • VEGAN • ONE POT

Oat bran cooks up quickly into a smooth, creamy, fiber-rich porridge—think of it as instant oats without the extra sugar and sodium. Cooking porridge with milk provides nutrition, and I use vanilla soy for the flavor and creaminess, but you can use any milk you prefer. (If you choose soy, look for a brand with no more than 8 grams of sugar per cup.) Eating soy-based foods has been linked to various health benefits, including lowered blood cholesterol. If you prefer, you can substitute almond or cashew milk, but you won't get as much protein—something most of us need to boost at breakfast.

Serves 2

Hands-on time: 5 min

Total time: 10 min

2 cups vanilla soy milk, plus more if needed

¾ cup oat bran

2 tablespoons natural peanut butter

2 teaspoons pure maple syrup

¼ teaspoon ground cinnamon

1 banana, sliced, divided

1 tablespoon hemp seeds, divided

1. Heat the soy milk in a large pot over high heat. Add the oat bran, peanut butter, maple syrup, and cinnamon, stirring as you go. When it starts to boil, turn the heat down to medium-low.

2. Cook for 2 minutes, stirring occasionally. Add more milk or water if you prefer a thinner consistency.

3. Divided the oatmeal between two bowls. Top each with half of the sliced banana and hemp seeds.

COOKING TIP: If you use cow's milk, cook more gently at a lower heat to avoid scorching.

PER SERVING: Calories: 354; Total Fat: 15g; Saturated Fat: 2g; Cholesterol: 0mg; Sodium: 123mg; Carbohydrates: 54g; Fiber: 9g; Added Sugars: 9g; Protein: 18g; Potassium: 861mg; Vitamin K: 5mcg

APPLE-PECAN OATMEAL

DASH • MEDITERRANEAN • VEGAN • ONE POT

Oatmeal is like a blank canvas, ready for you to dress it up with whatever fruit, nuts, seeds, and seasonings you're in the mood for. This is one of my family's favorite combinations. Instead of dried cherries, feel free to use dried cranberries, raisins, walnuts, or almonds if that's what you have on hand. It's all good!

Serves 2

Hands-on time: 10 min

Total time: 15 min

1½ cups vanilla soy milk

⅔ cup old-fashioned oats

2 small apples

2 tablespoons ground flaxseed, divided

½ teaspoon ground cinnamon, divided

⅓ cup roughly chopped pecans, divided

2 tablespoons dried cherries, divided

1. Heat the soy milk and oats in a medium pot over high heat. When the milk starts to bubble, turn it down to medium-low and simmer.

2. Meanwhile, core and dice the apples. Add them to the pot as you go.

3. When the oats and apples are done to your liking, after about 10 minutes, divide the oatmeal between two bowls. Top each with half of the flaxseed and cinnamon, then half of the pecans and cherries.

SUBSTITUTION TIP: If you prefer, use cow's milk, but heat it more gently.

FLAVOR BOOST: Add a pinch of ground cardamom or nutmeg or, for a touch of sweetness, a little brown sugar or pure maple syrup.

PER SERVING: Calories: 420; Total Fat: 20g; Saturated Fat: 2g; Cholesterol: 0mg; Sodium: 92mg; Carbohydrates: 56g; Fiber: 11g; Added Sugars: 8g; Protein: 11g; Potassium: 633mg; Vitamin K: 8mcg

CREAMY BLUEBERRY QUINOA PORRIDGE

DASH • MEDITERRANEAN • VEGETARIAN

Mix things up at breakfast with quinoa for a change! Some recipes recommend rinsing quinoa to wash away the bitter-tasting natural coating (saponin) that keeps insects away from the plant. But most quinoa sold today has been pre-rinsed, so check the package. You can probably save yourself a step.

Serves 2

Hands-on time: 10 min

Total time: 15 min

½ cup uncooked quinoa

1 cup 1% milk

½ cup water

1 cup Blueberry-Chia Jam (page 184), divided

2 tablespoons oat bran

⅓ cup chopped walnuts, divided

2 teaspoons pure maple syrup (optional), divided

1. Heat the quinoa, milk, and water in a medium pot over medium-high heat. When it starts to simmer, turn the heat to low, cover, and cook for 13 minutes (set a timer).

2. Meanwhile, reheat the chia jam in a small pot or in the microwave.

3. When the timer rings, add the oat bran to the quinoa, cover, and simmer for another 5 minutes.

4. Divide the porridge between two bowls. Top each with half of the chia jam, walnuts, and a drizzle of maple syrup (if using).

SUBSTITUTION TIP: If you don't have oat bran, substitute old-fashioned oats, adding them to the quinoa in step 1.

INGREDIENT TIP: The heart-healthy fats in walnuts and other nuts can become rancid quickly, so unless you're planning to use them in the next week or so, store nuts and seeds in the freezer to keep them tasting fresh.

PER SERVING: Calories: 423; Total Fat: 18g; Saturated Fat: 2g; Cholesterol: 6mg; Sodium: 58mg; Carbohydrates: 56g; Fiber: 8g; Added Sugars: 5g; Protein: 15g; Potassium: 608mg; Vitamin K: 14mcg

TOP THESE PANCAKES

Here's a great recipe to double for leftovers or to feed a hungry crowd. Serve topped with fruit, nuts, and/or seeds. Or try Better Butter (page 176), pure maple syrup, powdered sugar, or Blueberry-Chia Jam (page 184). You can get creative with the batter recipe, too. Try adding frozen berries, banana slices, or even canned pumpkin purée with a bit of pumpkin pie spice.

Serves 4 (2 to 3
pancakes per serving)

Hands-on time: 30 min

Total time: 30 min

1¼ cups 1% milk

1 cup quick oats

2 tablespoons canola or
sunflower oil, divided

2 large eggs

1 teaspoon vanilla extract

½ cup whole-wheat flour

1 tablespoon brown sugar

1 teaspoon baking powder

¼ teaspoon salt

1. Combine the milk, oats, 1 tablespoon of oil, eggs, and vanilla in a large bowl. Mix well. Stir in the flour, sugar, baking powder, and salt. Mix until the dry ingredients are just moistened.

2. Preheat a large skillet over medium-high heat. Add the remaining 1 tablespoon of oil, and tilt to coat.

3. Add ¼ cup of batter to the skillet for each pancake. Flip them when the tops are bubbly and the bottoms are golden, 2 to 3 minutes per side.

PER SERVING: Calories: 273; Total Fat: 12g; Saturated Fat: 2g; Cholesterol: 97mg; Sodium: 339mg; Carbohydrates: 32g; Fiber: 4g; Added Sugars: 3g; Protein: 10g; Potassium: 283mg; Vitamin K: 6mcg

MULTIGRAIN WAFFLES

DASH • VEGETARIAN

This surprisingly easy breakfast is always a hit with brunch guests. I like to offer a variety of toppings: chopped or sliced fruit, nuts, seeds, Blueberry-Chia Jam (page 184), pure maple syrup, and even peanut butter. This is portioned to pair with a protein-rich food, so you can round out the meal with Greek yogurt or a wedge of Spinach and Feta Frittata (page 50). Add a teaspoon of ground cinnamon to the batter, if you like. If you don't have a waffle iron, you can also make these into pancakes. Make the batter as directed then follow the cooking instructions for Top These Pancakes (page 45).

Serves 4 (1 small waffle per serving)

Hands-on time: 15 min

Total time: 20 min

¾ cup whole-wheat flour

¼ cup ground flaxseed

3 tablespoons rolled oats

2 tablespoons unsalted sunflower seeds

1½ teaspoons baking powder

1½ teaspoons brown sugar

¼ teaspoon salt

1 cup 1% milk

2 tablespoons canola or sunflower oil

1 large egg

1. Preheat a waffle iron.

2. Mix the flour, flaxseed, oats, sunflower seeds, baking powder, brown sugar, and salt in a large bowl. Add the milk, oil, and egg. Mix until just moistened.

3. Cover your waffle iron area with batter. Cook until golden and crisp (about 5 minutes for most waffle irons).

4. Serve immediately so the waffles are crisp and hot. If that's not possible, keep them warm directly on the rack in a 175°F oven.

SUBSTITUTION TIP: Make these waffles vegan with a plant-based milk and a "flax egg"—mix 1 tablespoon ground flaxseed with 3 tablespoons warm water and let sit for a few minutes.

LEFTOVERS: If you have a hungry crowd or want leftovers, double the recipe. Just reheat the waffles briefly in a toaster or oven.

PER SERVING: Calories: 264; Total Fat: 15g; Saturated Fat: 2g; Cholesterol: 50mg; Sodium: 376mg; Carbohydrates: 27g; Fiber: 5g; Added Sugars: 2g; Protein: 9g; Potassium: 298mg; Vitamin K: 6mcg

SOUTHWEST BREAKFAST TOFU

DASH • MEDITERRANEAN • VEGAN

Who says vegetables can't be part of a delicious breakfast? If the ones suggested here are not in season, try mushrooms or kale or any of your favorite veggies. Enjoy with Roasted Sweet Potatoes (page 68) or whole-grain toast or with Fresh Tomato Salsa (page 182) or hot sauce on top, for an extra kick. As in many recipes that use tofu, it's drained first to remove some of the water.

Serves 2

Hands-on time: 20 min

Total time: 20 min

1 (1-pound) block medium-firm tofu

¼ red onion

1 red bell pepper

1 tablespoon extra-virgin olive oil

1 teaspoon reduced-sodium tamari

1 tablespoon nutritional yeast

2 teaspoons Salt-Free Southwest Seasoning Mix (page 175) or Mrs. Dash, plus more if needed

⅛ to ¼ teaspoon salt (optional)

4 cups spinach

1 avocado, peeled, pitted, and diced (optional)

1. Drain the tofu, then cut through its equator to make two flat blocks. Wrap them in a couple of layers of clean kitchen towel or paper towel for at least 5 minutes. (It doesn't need to be pressed completely dry as in some other recipes.)

2. Meanwhile, chop the onion and seed and thinly slice the red pepper.

3. Heat the oil in a large, nonstick skillet on medium-high heat. When hot, turn it down to medium and cook the onion and pepper until soft, 4 to 5 minutes, stirring occasionally.

4. While that's cooking, mix the tamari, nutritional yeast, Southwest seasoning, and ⅛ teaspoon of salt in a small bowl.

5. When the onion and pepper are ready, add the spinach to the pan. Turn the heat down to medium-low, and cover for 1 minute to steam. Transfer the veggies to a bowl, and cover to keep warm.

→

6. Add the tofu and the tamari mixture to the pan, and mix well to combine. Use a wooden spoon to crumble the tofu. Taste and add another ⅛ teaspoon of salt or more Southwest seasoning, if needed.

7. Return the vegetables to the pan, and mix just a little. Top with the avocado (if using).

INGREDIENT TIPS: Tamari is similar to soy sauce, but with a richer, less salty flavor and usually no wheat, which is helpful for people who can't eat gluten. You'll find it near the soy sauce. Nutritional yeast is a nutrient-rich inactive yeast with a cheesy, nutty flavor. You can find it in the natural food aisle or in health food stores. Substitute grated Parmesan cheese if you like.

PER SERVING: Calories: 359; Total Fat: 26g; Saturated Fat: 4g; Cholesterol: 0mg; Sodium: 485mg; Carbohydrates: 16g; Fiber: 8g; Added Sugars: 0g; Protein: 21g; Potassium, 1,170mg; Vitamin K: 316mcg

CALIFORNIA SCRAMBLED EGGS AND VEGGIES

DASH • VEGETARIAN

Eggs aren't just for breakfast. This would make a satisfying lunch, too, or even a light supper. If you can't find or don't like arugula, use spinach instead. Serve with a slice of whole-grain toast—which you can spread with the avocado. Avocados might be high in fat, but it's a heart-healthy fat! They're also rich in fiber and vitamin E.

Serves 2

Hands-on time: 15 min

Total time: 15 min

4 large eggs

Pinch salt

Freshly ground
black pepper

2 teaspoons Better Butter
(page 176) or 1 teaspoon
extra-virgin olive oil plus
1 teaspoon unsalted butter

Handful of arugula
leaves, chopped

8 cherry tomatoes, halved

¼ cup chopped Simple
Roasted Peppers (page 61)
or jarred roasted red
peppers (optional)

1 avocado, peeled, pitted,
and diced

1. Crack the eggs into a large bowl. Season with salt and pepper, and whisk well.

2. In a large, nonstick skillet, melt the Better Butter over medium-low heat. When it starts to froth, add the arugula and sauté for a minute. Slide the arugula out of the pan and onto a plate.

3. Pour the eggs into the pan, and stir occasionally to scramble. When the eggs are almost done, sprinkle in the tomatoes, wilted arugula, and red pepper (if using). Don't stir. Put the lid on the pan, and cook for 1 more minute.

4. Top with the avocado.

FLAVOR BOOST: Take this dish to Baja California with a spoonful of diced Anaheim (mild) or jalapeño (spicier) peppers. Or try topping the eggs with crumbled goat cheese, chopped fresh basil, and minced, oil-packed sun-dried tomatoes.

PER SERVING: Calories: 315; Total Fat: 24g; Saturated Fat: 6g; Cholesterol: 377mg; Sodium: 393mg; Carbohydrates: 11g; Fiber: 6g; Added Sugars: 0g; Protein: 15g; Potassium: 681mg; Vitamin K: 32mcg

SPINACH AND FETA FRITTATA

DASH • VEGETARIAN

Frittata is like quiche without the pastry crust. Once you get the technique down, you can vary the ingredients depending on what you have on hand. For example, use roasted red peppers from a jar or ones you've roasted yourself, which will likely be much lower in sodium (see Simple Roasted Peppers, page 61). Or diced fresh peppers work well, too. It's delicious served on a piece of whole-grain toast with a light salad or fruit on the side. Leftovers are useful on weekday mornings.

Serves 4

Hands-on time: 15 min

Total time: 30 min

2 tablespoons extra-virgin olive oil

½ cup finely chopped onions

8 large eggs

¼ teaspoon black pepper

3 cups spinach, roughly chopped

½ cup roughly chopped Simple Roasted Peppers (page 61) or jarred roasted red peppers

⅓ cup crumbled feta cheese

1. Preheat the oven to 350°F.

2. Heat the oil in an 8- to 10-inch oven-safe skillet over medium-high heat. When hot, add the onion. Cook, stirring, until softened, about 5 minutes.

3. Meanwhile, in a large bowl, whisk together the eggs and pepper.

4. Add the spinach to the skillet, cover, and cook until slightly wilted, 1 to 2 minutes. Stir in the red peppers and cook for 1 to 2 minutes more. Lower the heat to medium, and add the eggs. Stir briefly to combine. Sprinkle the feta cheese on top.

5. Slide the skillet into the oven. Bake until the eggs are just set, about 15 minutes.

COOKING TIP: If you don't have an oven-safe skillet, just transfer the mixture to a baking dish. It will take a bit longer to cook.

PER SERVING: Calories: 254; Total Fat: 19g; Saturated Fat: 6g; Cholesterol: 383mg; Sodium: 418mg; Carbohydrates: 5g; Fiber: 1g; Added Sugars: 0g; Protein: 15g; Potassium: 280mg; Vitamin K: 95mcg

BREAKFAST VEGGIE BURRITO

DASH • VEGETARIAN

This burrito feels like a weekend treat but is easy enough to fuel you through a busy weekday morning. Enjoy with an orange and salsa, Greek yogurt, or sour cream. For an extra boost of flavor, add fresh cilantro or a sprinkle of Salt-Free Southwest Seasoning Mix (page 175) or Mrs. Dash.

Serves 2

Hands-on time: 15 min

Total time: 15 min

3 large eggs

2 (10-inch) whole-grain tortillas

4 thin slices Cheddar cheese

2 cups spinach, divided

1 medium tomato, chopped, divided

2 tablespoons Fresh Tomato Salsa (page 182) or lower-sodium store-bought salsa, divided

1 tablespoon extra-virgin olive oil

1. Crack the eggs into a large bowl. Beat gently with a fork.

2. Set out two plates, and place a tortilla on each. Line 2 cheese slices down the middle of each tortilla. Top each with half of the spinach, then half of the tomato and salsa.

3. Heat the olive oil in a nonstick skillet over medium heat, tilting to coat the pan. Add the eggs, and stir occasionally until they're scrambled.

4. When the eggs are done, spoon them on top of the tomatoes and salsa.

5. Gently fold in the sides of the tortillas, and roll them up.

6. Place the burritos, seam-side down, in the skillet (wiped clean if necessary), cover, and warm gently for 2 to 3 minutes over medium heat. Keep a close eye so you don't burn them!

INGREDIENT TIP: Check the labels when you buy salsa. Some have much less sodium than others, and some even have added sugar.

COOKING TIP: Just 30 seconds in the microwave will warm these burritos and get you going faster.

PER SERVING: Calories: 471; Total Fat: 27g; Saturated Fat: 8g; Cholesterol: 300mg; Sodium: 627mg; Carbohydrates: 35g; Fiber: 8g; Added Sugars: 0g; Protein: 22g; Potassium: 631mg; Vitamin K: 159mcg

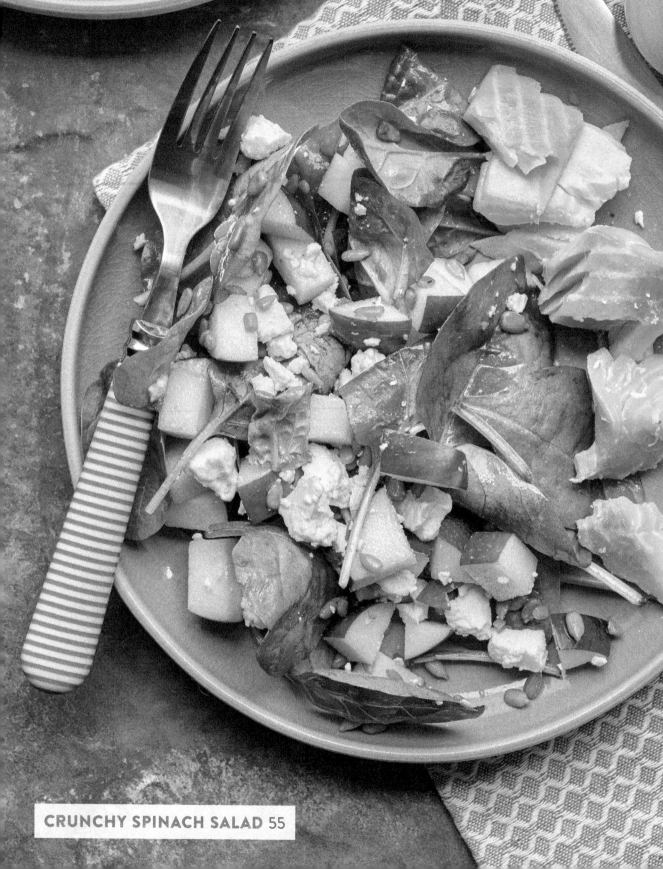

CRUNCHY SPINACH SALAD 55

CHAPTER THREE

SALADS, STARTERS, AND SIDE DISHES

CLASSIC CAPRESE SALAD

DASH • MEDITERRANEAN • VEGETARIAN • NO-COOK

This tomato and mozzarella cheese salad is an elegant summer classic—great for impressing guests. It's best with in-season tomatoes and good-quality olive oil and balsamic vinegar. Add fresh whole-grain bread, and you have a simple dinner for those days when it's too hot to cook. I suggest an approximate amount of kosher salt here, but trust your palate. Some fresh mozzarella has nearly no salt, some has a little. Some tomatoes are bursting with flavor, some less so. You may need a little more salt than the recipe calls for to make this dish sing. Sprinkle it evenly over the dish with your fingers for the most control.

Serves 4

Hands-on time: 15 min

Total time: 15 min

6 small tomatoes

8 ounces fresh
mozzarella cheese

¼ teaspoon kosher salt,
plus more if needed

Freshly ground black
pepper (optional)

⅓ cup torn fresh
basil leaves

2 tablespoons extra-virgin
olive oil

2 tablespoons
balsamic vinegar

1. Use a serrated knife to cut the tomatoes and cheese into ¼-inch slices. You should have about the same number of each. If not, cut some pieces in half. so you do

2. Arrange the tomatoes and cheese on a serving platter in alternating slices.

3. Sprinkle with salt and pepper (if using). Spread the basil over the salad. Drizzle with the olive oil and balsamic vinegar. Taste and adjust the seasoning.

FLAVOR BOOST: Try this recipe with goat cheese instead of mozzarella, dried oregano and fresh arugula instead of basil, balsamic glaze instead of vinegar, and roasted red peppers instead of tomatoes.

PER SERVING: Calories: 252; Total Fat: 21g; Saturated Fat: 9g; Cholesterol: 40mg; Sodium: 159mg; Carbohydrates: 7g; Fiber: 2g; Added Sugars: 0g; Protein: 11g; Potassium: 338mg; Vitamin K: 23mcg

CRUNCHY SPINACH SALAD

DASH • MEDITERRANEAN • VEGETARIAN • 5-INGREDIENT • NO-COOK

Salted sunflower seeds add only about 50 mg of sodium per serving, so use them if you prefer. Make this salad into a meal by adding a can of chickpeas (rinsed and drained) or topping the salad with slices of cooked chicken, such as Pan-Seared Chicken (page 120). You can prepare the salad while the chicken is cooking.

Serves 4

Hands-on time: 20 min

Total time: 20 min
(including making the
vinaigrette)

1 (5-ounce) package
spinach (about 6 cups
loosely packed)

1 apple

¼ cup unsalted
sunflower seeds

¼ cup crumbled
feta cheese

¼ cup Red Wine Vinaigrette
(page 178)

1. Trim any large stems from the spinach, and tear any large leaves. Core and chop the apple.

2. In a large bowl, combine the spinach, apple, sunflower seeds, and feta cheese. Drizzle on the vinaigrette, and toss to coat.

COOKING TIP: Start with prewashed baby spinach for a super-fast salad. It's sold in the produce department.

PER SERVING: Calories: 174; Total Fat: 14g; Saturated Fat: 3g; Cholesterol: 8mg; Sodium: 191mg; Carbohydrates: 11g; Fiber: 3g; Added Sugars: 1g; Protein: 4g; Potassium: 327mg; Vitamin K: 177mcg

AWESOME ARUGULA SALAD

DASH • MEDITERRANEAN • VEGETARIAN

Arugula, also known as rocket, has a peppery flavor and is a potent source of nitrate, which may help keep blood pressure in check. This salad is outrageously easy and delicious. Substitute whatever nuts or seeds you have on hand. Lightly toasting raw nuts and seeds is optional but greatly enhances their flavor and texture. Commercially roasted nuts and seeds pale in comparison flavor-wise but are fine health-wise.

Serves 4

Hands-on time: 15 min

Total time: 15 min

¼ cup unsalted raw sunflower seeds

5 ounces arugula

1 cup grape or cherry tomatoes, halved

2 tablespoons extra-virgin olive oil

1 tablespoon rice vinegar

¼ cup grated Parmesan cheese

1 avocado, peeled, pitted, and sliced (optional)

¼ cup dried cranberries (optional)

Freshly ground black pepper (optional)

1. Preheat the oven to 350°F.

2. Spread the sunflower seeds on a rimmed baking sheet, and put them in the oven. Shake after 5 minutes, check after another 3 minutes, and take them out when they look golden and smell nutty, usually no more than 12 minutes total. Remove from the pan to cool.

3. Toss the arugula, tomatoes, oil, vinegar, and cheese in a large bowl.

4. Top with the toasted sunflower seeds, sliced avocado, cranberries, and pepper (if using).

SUBSTITUTION TIP: For a vegan alternative, skip the Parmesan and double the seeds. After toasting them, mix in a bowl with 2 teaspoons nutritional yeast, 1½ teaspoons extra-virgin olive oil, and a pinch of salt.

PER SERVING: Calories: 232; Total Fat: 18g; Saturated Fat: 3g; Cholesterol: 4mg; Sodium: 158mg; Carbohydrates: 17g; Fiber: 5g; Added Sugars: 0g; Protein: 5g; Potassium: 492mg; Vitamin K: 54mcg

QUICK KALE CAESAR SALAD

DASH • MEDITERRANEAN • VEGETARIAN • NO-COOK • PORTABLE

Prewashed baby kale typically comes in 5-ounce packages. You can substitute one bunch of regular kale; remove the tough stems and finely chop the leaves. Put them in a large bowl with a tablespoon or so of olive oil, and massage for a minute to soften the leaves before proceeding with the recipe. In fact, this dish gets even better if it can sit for 10 minutes after tossing with the dressing but before adding the Parmesan crisps to soften the kale. This simple salad goes well with Rosemary-Lemon Salmon (page 112) or Pan-Seared Chicken (page 120).

Serves 4

Hands-on time: 15 min

Total time: 15 min

For the dressing

2 tablespoons extra-virgin olive oil, plus more if needed

2 tablespoons mayonnaise

1 tablespoon freshly squeezed lemon juice

1 tablespoon red wine vinegar

1 teaspoon Dijon mustard

1 small garlic clove, minced

⅛ teaspoon kosher salt

For the salad

1 (5-ounce) package prewashed baby kale

2 tablespoons grated Parmesan cheese

¼ cup Parmesan crisps (optional)

1. In a large bowl, whisk together the oil, mayonnaise, lemon juice, vinegar, mustard, garlic, and salt.

2. Add the kale and toss well with the dressing, then add the Parmesan cheese and toss again. If needed, add a bit more oil, so it's not dry.

3. Top with Parmesan crisps (if using).

INGREDIENT TIP: Parmesan crisps are like small crackers, but they're made of nothing more than baked aged Parmesan cheese. They're delicious and more nutritious than croutons, but similarly high in sodium, so use just a few. Find them in the deli section or near the condiments.

FLAVOR BOOST: For more fiber, try topping the salad with roasted chickpeas. Look for them where you buy nuts and seeds.

PER SERVING: Calories: 156; Total Fat: 14g; Saturated Fat: 3g; Cholesterol: 8mg; Sodium: 242mg; Carbohydrates: 4g; Fiber: 1g; Added Sugars: 0g; Protein: 4g; Potassium: 191mg; Vitamin K: 266mcg

ZESTY CHICKPEA AND TOMATO SALAD

DASH • MEDITERRANEAN • VEGETARIAN • NO-COOK • PORTABLE

This is one of my favorite recipes for chickpeas because it's so easy and so delicious! There are lots of ways to play with this basic salad. Add ground cumin, diced bell pepper, or garlic. Pair it with a crusty whole-grain roll and an orange for a light lunch, or dish up a cup of it for a satisfying snack. Rinsing canned beans removes only about 40 percent of the sodium, so it's still worth it to look for a lower-sodium brand—or cook them up from scratch, if you can. If you're using regular canned chickpeas in this recipe, rinse them very well and reduce the salt to ⅛ teaspoon.

Serves 4

Hands-on time: 15 min

Total time: 15 min

1 (15-ounce) can no-salt-added chickpeas, rinsed and drained

2 plum tomatoes, chopped

1 cup chopped fresh cilantro

¼ cup finely chopped red onion

Zest and juice of ½ lemon (about 1½ tablespoons juice)

2 teaspoons dried cumin

1 tablespoon extra-virgin olive oil

2 teaspoons honey

¼ teaspoon kosher salt

Freshly ground black pepper

Combine the chickpeas, tomatoes, cilantro, onion, lemon zest and juice, cumin, oil, honey, salt, and pepper in a large bowl, and toss well to mix.

INGREDIENT TIP: Zest is the thin, colored, flavorful outer layer of a citrus fruit, such as lemon. It comes in handy when you want to add a little zing without much salt. A fine grater is the easiest way to get it—just be careful not to grate the bitter white pith beneath the zest. Use as much or as little as you like.

PER SERVING: Calories: 163; Total Fat: 4g; Saturated Fat: 0g; Cholesterol: 0mg; Sodium: 150mg; Carbohydrates: 23g; Fiber: 5g; Added Sugars: 3g; Protein: 6g; Potassium: 299mg; Vitamin K: 17mcg

PEAR AND PUMPKIN SEED SALAD

DASH • MEDITERRANEAN • VEGETARIAN • NO-COOK

This recipe is adapted from one shared by my friend Heidi nearly 20 years ago. The pears are a great source of cholesterol-lowering soluble fiber, and the Parmesan cheese and crunchy pumpkin seeds keep people coming back for seconds. Shelled pumpkin seeds are sometimes called pepitas. People often avoid salted nuts and seeds, but because the salt is on the surface, they can add a lot of taste without much sodium. The salted pumpkin seeds in this salad add only about 25 mg sodium per serving—not much in the grand scheme of things. Add them just before serving so they stay crunchy.

Serves 4

Hands-on time: 20 min

Total time: 20 min

For the dressing

3 tablespoons extra-virgin olive oil

2 teaspoons Dijon mustard

2 teaspoons cooking sherry

2 teaspoons red wine vinegar

For the salad

1 head butter lettuce, torn into pieces

2 Bosc pears, cored and cut into bite-size pieces

¼ cup salted shelled pumpkin seeds

½ cup grated Parmesan cheese

Freshly ground black pepper (optional)

1. In a large bowl, whisk together the oil, mustard, sherry, and vinegar.

2. Add the lettuce and pears, and toss well to coat with the dressing.

3. Top with the pumpkin seeds, Parmesan cheese, and a grind of pepper, if you like.

SUBSTITUTION TIP: Use green leaf lettuce if you can't find butter lettuce.

PER SERVING: Calories: 244; Total Fat: 17g; Saturated Fat: 4g; Cholesterol: 7mg; Sodium: 219mg; Carbohydrates: 18g; Fiber: 4g; Added Sugars: 0g; Protein: 7g; Potassium: 291mg; Vitamin K: 53mcg

ORANGE AND AVOCADO GREEN SALAD

DASH • MEDITERRANEAN • VEGETARIAN

This light salad pairs well with salmon, chicken, or white beans. Add a cup of cooked quinoa or hearty sprouted-grain toast to make it a meal. Slice some radishes into the salad for an extra pop of flavor. And make it even easier by using a bag of prewashed baby romaine lettuce.

Serves 4

Hands-on time: 25 min

Total time: 25 min

¼ cup shelled pistachios

1 large orange

2 tablespoons extra-virgin olive oil

2 tablespoons plain yogurt

2 teaspoons freshly squeezed lemon juice (about ½ small lemon)

2 teaspoons pure maple syrup

¼ teaspoon kosher salt

Freshly ground black pepper

1 head butter, green leaf, or red leaf lettuce, torn into bite-size pieces

1 avocado, peeled, pitted, and chopped

1. Preheat the oven to 350°F.

2. Spread the pistachios on a rimmed baking sheet and transfer to the oven. Shake after 5 minutes, check after another 3 minutes, and take them out when they look golden and smell nutty, usually no more than 12 minutes total. Remove from the pan to cool. When cool, chop them roughly.

3. Cut the orange in half. Squeeze the juice from one half into a large bowl for the dressing. Add the olive oil, yogurt, lemon juice, maple syrup, salt, and a grind of pepper; mix well.

4. Peel the other half of the orange, then cut the flesh into bite-size pieces. Add the lettuce, orange pieces, avocado, and pistachios to the bowl with the dressing, and toss well.

SUBSTITUTION TIP: Make this vegan by substituting tahini for the yogurt. Use walnuts or almonds instead of pistachios, if that's easier.

PER SERVING: Calories: 198; Total Fat: 16g; Saturated Fat: 2g; Cholesterol: 0mg; Sodium: 165mg; Carbohydrates: 13g; Fiber: 4g; Added Sugars: 2g; Protein: 4g; Potassium: 436mg; Vitamin K: 54mcg

SIMPLE ROASTED PEPPERS

DASH • MEDITERRANEAN • VEGAN

Enjoy these roasted peppers as a quick side dish, or toss them with pasta and goat cheese. The recipe calls for four, but really, you can roast as many as you like and keep them in an airtight container in the refrigerator for about a week. Jarred roasted peppers from the store are peeled after roasting, but for a quick weeknight meal, you don't have to bother. This technique also works with mushrooms, zucchini, asparagus, carrots, broccoli, cauliflower, and other vegetables.

Serves 4

Hands-on time: 10 min

Total time: 25 min

4 red, yellow, and orange bell peppers, seeded and sliced

1 red onion, sliced (optional)

2 tablespoons canola or sunflower oil

¼ teaspoon salt (optional)

Freshly ground black pepper (optional)

1. Preheat the oven to 400°F.

2. Combine the peppers and onion (if using) in a large bowl. Add the oil and toss gently.

3. Spread out the peppers on one or two rimmed baking sheets. Make sure they're not too crowded, or they'll steam instead of roast.

4. Roast the peppers for 15 minutes, then toss them and roast for 5 minutes more, until they're done to your liking. Charred spots are fine—even desirable. Season with salt and pepper, if you want.

FLAVOR BOOST: After roasting, stir in some minced garlic, red wine vinegar, balsamic vinegar, fresh oregano, or fresh thyme.

PER SERVING: Calories: 110; Total Fat: 7g; Saturated Fat: 1g; Cholesterol: 0mg; Sodium: 151mg; Carbohydrates: 10g; Fiber: 3g; Added Sugars: 0g; Protein: 1g; Potassium: 291mg; Vitamin K: 11mcg

CREAMY TOMATO-BASIL SOUP

DASH • MEDITERRANEAN • VEGAN

This tomato soup is basic comfort food, and much lower in sodium than what you'll find in a can or at a restaurant. Tofu adds protein and healthy fats, but if you prefer light cream, use a little of that instead, or just enjoy it as is. If you don't have fresh basil, look for basil stir-in paste in the produce department. It tastes great in this soup.

Serves 8 (1 cup per serving)

Hands-on time: 15 min

Total time: 25 min

1 tablespoon extra-virgin olive oil

¼ large onion, peeled and roughly chopped

1 carrot, peeled and sliced

1 celery stalk, sliced

1 garlic clove, minced

2 teaspoons dried oregano

1 (28-ounce) can no-salt-added whole tomatoes

1 cup reduced-sodium vegetable broth

1 (10-ounce) block soft tofu, drained (optional)

¼ teaspoon salt (optional)

Freshly ground black pepper (optional)

¼ cup finely chopped fresh basil

1. Heat the oil in a large pot over medium-high heat. When hot, add the onion, carrot, celery, and garlic. Sauté for 4 to 5 minutes, until the onion is soft.

2. Add the oregano, and stir for a minute. Add the tomatoes with their juice and the broth. Bring to a boil, then lower the heat and simmer for 10 minutes.

3. If desired, transfer a cup of the soup to a blender or food processor. Add the tofu, and blend well. Return this mixture to the pot, and stir it into the rest of the soup.

4. Season with salt and pepper, if you like. Ladle into bowls, and top with the basil.

FLAVOR BOOST: Garnish with toasted pumpkin seeds or slivered almonds.

PER SERVING: Calories: 95; Total Fat: 5g; Saturated Fat: 1g; Cholesterol: 0mg; Sodium: 135mg; Carbohydrates: 6g; Fiber: 3g; Added Sugars: 0g; Protein: 8g; Potassium: 254mg; Vitamin K: 12mcg

BLACK BEAN AND SALSA SOUP

This simple soup comes together in no time. Enjoy it with a whole-wheat roll and you've got a light, simple meal loaded with both veggies and flavor. Or top each bowl with some chopped avocado or homemade Baked Tortilla Chips (page 155). If you're using store-bought salsa, look for a brand with 130 mg or less of sodium per 2-tablespoon serving.

Serves 6 (1 cup per serving)

Hands-on time: 10 min

Total time: 10 min

1½ cups reduced-sodium vegetable broth

1 (15-ounce) can no-salt-added black beans, rinsed and drained

½ cup frozen corn kernels

½ cup Fresh Tomato Salsa (page 182) or lower-sodium store-bought salsa

1½ cups chopped fresh or frozen broccoli

1½ teaspoons freshly squeezed lime juice, divided

¾ cup shredded Cheddar cheese, divided

2 scallions, thinly sliced, divided

Dash hot sauce, divided (optional)

1. In a large pot, combine the broth, black beans, corn, and salsa. Bring to a boil over high heat.

2. Add the broccoli, and cook for 2 to 4 minutes (longer for fresh broccoli); remove the pot from the heat as soon as the broccoli is tender—it will continue to cook in the hot liquid.

3. Ladle the soup into bowls. To each serving, add ¼ teaspoon of lime juice, 3 tablespoons of shredded Cheddar, a sprinkle of scallions, and a dash of hot sauce, if desired.

SUBSTITUTION TIP: Make this soup vegan by skipping the cheese and topping the soup with chopped toasted pecans or pumpkin seeds.

PER SERVING: Calories: 166; Total Fat: 6g; Saturated Fat: 3g; Cholesterol: 16mg; Sodium: 245mg; Carbohydrates: 18g; Fiber: 6g; Added Sugars: 0g; Protein: 10g; Potassium: 420mg; Vitamin K: 39mcg

UMAMI MUSHROOMS

DASH • MEDITERRANEAN • VEGAN • 5-INGREDIENT • ONE POT

Mushrooms might not be brightly colored, but they are nutritious—they're a good source of selenium, potassium, and B vitamins. They're also one of the best vegetable sources of umami, the fifth taste, which is responsible for the savory deliciousness associated with aged meats and cheeses. Umami is also found in tamari and balsamic vinegar, so this combination is a great way to add flavor to lean meat or steamed vegetables. Use any mushrooms you like—or a combo—but the dish will have even more flavor if you use cremini or portobello mushrooms.

Serves 2

Hands-on time: 15 min

Total time: 15 min

8 ounces white button, cremini, or portobello mushrooms

2 tablespoons extra-virgin olive oil

1 tablespoon balsamic vinegar

2 teaspoons reduced-sodium tamari

1 garlic clove, minced

1. Rinse the mushrooms, then pat them dry with a paper towel. Trim them only if the ends look tough, and cut them into thick slices.

2. Preheat a heavy skillet over medium-high heat. Add the oil to pan. When the oil is shimmering, add the mushrooms and toss to coat. Cook, stirring only occasionally, for 7 to 10 minutes, until any water released by the mushrooms has evaporated and they're golden brown. If they start to brown too quickly, turn down the heat.

3. Turn the heat down to medium-low. Add the balsamic vinegar and tamari, and sauté until dry. Add the garlic, and sauté for 1 minute.

FLAVOR BOOST: Add even more savory flavor with cooking sherry or dry white wine and fresh or dry oregano, thyme, tarragon, or chives. Add them in step 3, along with the vinegar and tamari.

PER SERVING: Calories: 157; Total Fat: 14g; Saturated Fat: 2g; Cholesterol: 0mg; Sodium: 200mg; Carbohydrates: 6g; Fiber: 1g; Added Sugars: 0g; Protein: 4g; Potassium: 394mg; Vitamin K: 8mcg

PURÉED CARROTS AND GOAT CHEESE

DASH • MEDITERRANEAN • VEGETARIAN • 5-INGREDIENT

Don't let the talk about sugar in carrots scare you—the amount of sugar in a large carrot is about as much as in a handful of blueberries. Both are rich in antioxidants and can be part of a heart-healthy eating plan. This same preparation method also works well with cauliflower, sweet potatoes, and butternut squash. For a heartier dish, toss the purée with hot rotini pasta.

Serves 4

Hands-on time: 10 min

Total time: 25 min

2 pounds baby carrots

½ cup crumbled goat cheese

1. Put the carrots in a large pot, and pour in enough water to just about but not quite cover them. Bring to a boil over high heat, then turn down the heat, cover, and simmer for 20 minutes. The carrots should be quite tender.

2. Pour about half of the cooking water into a glass measuring cup or a bowl. Carefully transfer the carrots and remaining cooking water to a food processor or blender. If using a blender, remove the center cap from the lid and hold a dish towel over the hole while blending to prevent steam from building up.

3. Purée until the mixture is very smooth. Add some of the reserved cooking water if needed to make it creamy.

4. Add the goat cheese, and purée until well blended.

SUBSTITUTION TIP: Make this dish vegan by replacing the goat cheese with a drizzle of flavorful extra-virgin olive oil and a pinch of salt.

PER SERVING: Calories: 142; Total Fat: 5g; Saturated Fat: 4g; Cholesterol: 13mg; Sodium: 253mg; Carbohydrates: 19g; Fiber: 7g; Added Sugars: 0g; Protein: 6g; Potassium: 551mg; Vitamin K: 22mcg

SAUTÉED SPINACH WITH PUMPKIN SEEDS

DASH • MEDITERRANEAN • VEGETARIAN

Add a vegetable to your dinner entrée in minutes with this simple side dish. Use a 5-ounce bag of prewashed spinach, and you can make the whole thing in under 10 minutes. Toasting the pumpkin seeds is optional, but it brings out their nutty flavor and gives them a nice crunch. Stir in a tablespoon or two of Walnut Pesto (page 181) for an extra splash of flavor.

Serves 2

Hands-on time: 15 min

Total time: 20 min

2 tablespoons raw shelled pumpkin seeds

2 teaspoons extra-virgin olive oil

1 teaspoon balsamic vinegar

1 teaspoon water

1 bunch spinach, large stems removed

2 tablespoons crumbled goat cheese or feta cheese

Freshly ground black pepper (optional)

1. Preheat the oven to 350°F.

2. Spread the pumpkin seeds on a rimmed baking sheet, and transfer them to the oven. Shake after 5 minutes, check after another 3 minutes, and take them out when they look golden and smell nutty, usually no more than 12 minutes total. Remove from the pan to cool.

3. Heat the oil, vinegar, and water in a large skillet over medium-high heat. When it is hot, add the spinach. Cover and cook for a minute, then stir so the spinach gets coated with the oil and vinegar and just barely wilts, another minute or so.

4. Transfer to a serving dish, and sprinkle with the toasted pumpkin seeds and goat cheese. Top with black pepper, if desired.

SUBSTITUTION TIP: For a vegan dish, omit the cheese and top the spinach with a tablespoon or so of dried cranberries or dried cherries.

PER SERVING: Calories: 136; Total Fat: 11g; Saturated Fat: 3g; Cholesterol: 7mg; Sodium: 107mg; Carbohydrates: 5g; Fiber: 2g; Added Sugars: 0g; Protein: 7g; Potassium: 543mg; Vitamin K: 414mcg

LIFE-CHANGING ROASTED CAULIFLOWER

DASH • MEDITERRANEAN • VEGAN • 5-INGREDIENT • ONE POT

Not to be overly dramatic, but making crispy roasted cauliflower (and other vegetables) from frozen is life changing! You get more delicious vegetables with less prep time, expense, and food waste. Make sure you get frozen florets and not cauliflower "rice," and spread them out evenly on the baking sheet. Use two sheets if necessary, because if the vegetables are too close to each other when roasting, they'll end up steaming instead. This recipe also works well for frozen broccoli, butternut squash, and carrots.

Serves 2

Hands-on time: 10 min

Total time: 30 min

1 (12-ounce) bag frozen cauliflower florets (about 3 cups)

2 tablespoons canola or sunflower oil

¼ teaspoon kosher salt

½ teaspoon ground cumin (optional)

Freshly ground black pepper (optional)

1. Preheat the oven to 420°F. Line a rimmed baking sheet with parchment paper.

2. Put the cauliflower on the baking sheet, and toss gently with the oil, salt, cumin, and pepper (if using). Spread out the cauliflower in a single layer.

3. Roast the cauliflower for about 25 minutes, tossing every 10 minutes so it cooks evenly. Don't worry if it gets dark brown in spots—that's the best part.

FLAVOR BOOST: Skip the cumin and season with any or all of the following when the cauliflower comes out of the oven: more fresh black pepper, 1 tablespoon grated Parmesan cheese, 2 teaspoons freshly squeezed lemon juice, and/or the zest from the lemon.

PER SERVING: Calories: 166; Total Fat: 15g; Saturated Fat: 1g; Cholesterol: 0mg; Sodium: 282mg; Carbohydrates: 8g; Fiber: 4g; Added Sugars: 0g; Protein: 3g; Potassium: 328mg; Vitamin K: 35mcg

ROASTED SWEET POTATOES

DASH • MEDITERRANEAN • VEGAN • PORTABLE

This is a simple, crowd-pleasing side that takes only a few minutes of hands-on work. If you're in a hurry, just toss the potatoes with oil and a little salt and pepper and leave out all the other seasonings—they're still delicious. Or, try Salt-Free Southwest Seasoning Mix (page 175) instead. Jazz this up by roasting wedges of sweet onion along with the sweet potatoes. Leftovers are great for breakfast or lunch, even cold.

Serves 4

Hands-on time: 10 min

Total time: 30 min

2 large sweet potatoes, well scrubbed

2 tablespoons canola or sunflower oil

½ teaspoon garlic powder

½ teaspoon onion powder

½ teaspoon dried oregano

½ teaspoon paprika

¼ teaspoon kosher salt

Freshly ground black pepper

1. Preheat the oven to 425°F. Line two rimmed baking sheets with parchment paper.

2. Cut the sweet potatoes into ¾-inch chunks. Toss the potatoes with the oil and the garlic powder, onion powder, oregano, paprika, salt, and pepper in a large bowl. Divide the coated potato pieces between the prepared baking sheets, spreading them out in single layers and making sure they aren't crowded.

3. Cook for about 25 minutes, turning every 10 minutes or so.

COOKING TIP: The parchment paper helps keep the sweet potatoes from burning at this high temperature. Parchment is nonstick, compostable, and oven-safe up to 425°F. If you don't have parchment on hand, you can go without, but turn the temperature down to 400°F and give it a few extra minutes.

PER SERVING: Calories: 177; Total Fat: 7g; Saturated Fat: 1g; Cholesterol: 0mg; Sodium: 192mg; Carbohydrates: 27g; Fiber: 4g; Added Sugars: 0g; Protein: 2g; Potassium: 454mg; Vitamin K: 8mcg

HEARTY MASHED POTATOES

The trick to making heart-healthier mashed potatoes is to go easy on the butter and salt, but not so much that you no longer enjoy them! Everyone's preferences are different, so add salt to taste. Leave the skins on your potatoes to save time, add texture, and preserve the nutrients—fiber, vitamin C, potassium, and more. The Greek yogurt provides creaminess, much like sour cream, so you can use less butter. And nutritional yeast lends an earthy, cheese-like flavor.

Serves 4

Hands-on time: 10 min

Total time: 25 min

1½ pounds mini new potatoes

1 tablespoon extra-virgin olive oil

1 tablespoon unsalted butter

½ cup plain 2% Greek yogurt

1 tablespoon nutritional yeast (optional)

¼ teaspoon salt (optional)

Freshly ground black pepper (optional)

Snipped fresh chives, for garnish (optional)

1. Put the potatoes in a large pot, and pour in just enough water to cover them. Bring the water to a boil over high heat, then turn the heat down, cover, and simmer until the tip of a sharp knife slides easily into a potato, about 18 minutes.

2. Drain the potatoes, reserving the cooking water. Put the potatoes back in the pot, and turn the heat down to low. Use a potato masher to mash the potatoes with the olive oil and butter, then the yogurt. Add the reserved cooking water, ½ cup at a time, until the potatoes are as creamy as you like.

3. Using a wooden spoon, mix in the nutritional yeast, salt, and pepper (if using).

4. Taste, and adjust the seasonings. Top with snipped fresh chives, if you like, and another grind of black pepper.

SUBSTITUTION TIP: For a vegan dish, use a vegan buttery spread and skip the yogurt.

PER SERVING: Calories: 214; Total Fat: 7g; Saturated Fat: 3g; Cholesterol: 11mg; Sodium: 168mg; Carbohydrates: 32g; Fiber: 4g; Added Sugars: 0g; Protein: 7g; Potassium: 801mg; Vitamin K: 19mcg

SPAGHETTI SQUASH WITH WALNUTS AND PARMESAN

DASH • MEDITERRANEAN • VEGETARIAN • 5-INGREDIENT

Spaghetti squash is widely touted as a pasta substitute, but I think that does it a disservice. It's delicious in its own right, with a sweet, mild flavor. Whole spaghetti squash steams quickly in the microwave, but if your microwave or dish isn't large enough to hold both halves at once, you can do one and then the other. For a vegan variation, skip the cheese and use more nuts.

Serves 4

Hands-on time: 15 min

Total time: 30 min

1 small spaghetti squash

2 tablespoons extra-virgin olive oil

¼ cup chopped walnuts

1 garlic clove, minced

¼ cup grated Parmesan cheese, divided

1. Poke the squash a few times with a fork, then microwave on high for 3 to 4 minutes to soften. Don't microwave longer than 5 minutes, or the steam buildup may cause it to burst.

2. Carefully halve the squash lengthwise. Use a spoon to scrape out the seeds. Place the halves, cut-sides down, in a microwave-safe baking dish. Pour in ½ inch of water.

3. Microwave on high until you can easily pierce the squash with a fork, 8 to 12 minutes.

4. Meanwhile, warm the oil, walnuts, and garlic in a small saucepan over low heat.

5. When the squash is done and cool enough to handle, use a fork to loosen the spaghetti-like strands of flesh. Pile them into four bowls, and top each with a quarter of the garlic-infused oil, walnuts, and cheese.

FLAVOR BOOST: Top with a chopped tomato and fresh or dried basil. Or swap the toppings for Walnut Pesto (page 181), Mushroom Bolognese (page 137), or Roasted Tomato and Chicken Pasta (page 131).

PER SERVING: Calories: 228; Total Fat: 15g; Saturated Fat: 3g; Cholesterol: 3mg; Sodium: 124mg; Carbohydrates: 24g; Fiber: 5g; Added Sugars: 0g; Protein: 5g; Potassium: 388mg; Vitamin K: 7mcg

BRUSSELS SPROUTS AND PANCETTA

You might be surprised to see pancetta, Italian-style bacon, in a heart-healthy cookbook. Turns out that foods aren't "good" or "bad," "healthy" or "unhealthy." It's our overall dietary pattern that matters. Processed and fatty meats can be a part of a heart-healthy life—just in smaller amounts than is typical. Think of them as a flavoring, as in this recipe, or an occasional treat. Check the amounts of saturated fat and sodium in this dish—you'll see they aren't very high. Thanks to my bacon-loving sister, Tracy, for sharing this recipe.

Serves 4

Hands-on time: 25 min

Total time: 25 min

1 pound Brussels sprouts, trimmed and halved

1 onion, diced

½ cup cubed pancetta

3 garlic cloves, minced

1 teaspoon balsamic vinegar

¼ cup slivered almonds

⅛ teaspoon salt

Freshly ground black pepper

1. Pour an inch or so of water into a medium pot, and bring to a boil over medium-high heat. Add the Brussels sprouts, cover, and cook for 6 minutes.

2. Meanwhile, in a large, heavy skillet, sauté the onion and pancetta until the onion is transparent, 3 to 4 minutes. Add the garlic, balsamic vinegar, and almonds. Cook for another minute, then slide them out of the pan and onto a plate.

3. Use a slotted spoon to transfer the Brussels sprouts to the same skillet, cut-sides down, and sauté over medium-high heat for 5 to 7 minutes. When they start to get crisp, add the onion mixture and mix thoroughly. Season with salt and pepper.

SUBSTITUTION TIP: If you can't find pancetta, use four strips of regular bacon, chopped.

PER SERVING: Calories: 208; Total Fat: 14g; Saturated Fat: 4g; Cholesterol: 16mg; Sodium: 472mg; Carbohydrates: 15g; Fiber: 6g; Added Sugars: 0g; Protein: 9g; Potassium: 591mg; Vitamin K: 201mcg

LEMONY COUSCOUS TABBOULEH

DASH • MEDITERRANEAN • VEGAN • PORTABLE

A Lebanese family immigrated to Canada, and their kids started school with ours. I invited them to dinner and asked the mother what they would like. Surprisingly, she said tabbouleh! But when I served it, there were awkward whispers of, "Mama, this is not tabbouleh." Turns out that proper Lebanese tabbouleh is mostly fresh parsley and tomatoes, not grain like my version. Plus, I had thrown in chickpeas and feta cheese—not so authentic! We laughed about it, and she shared her favorite recipe, which I've adapted here. I use whole-wheat couscous because it's easier to find than the classic extra-fine bulgur. If you can find that, use it instead.

Serves 4

Hands-on time: 20 min

Total time: 20 min

1 tablespoon uncooked whole-wheat couscous

1½ tablespoons boiling water

4 cups fresh curly parsley (about 2 bunches), finely chopped

¼ cup finely chopped fresh mint

2 ripe tomatoes, finely chopped

2 scallions, finely sliced

¼ cup extra-virgin olive oil

Grated zest and juice of ½ lemon (about 1½ tablespoons juice)

¼ teaspoon salt

¼ teaspoon freshly ground black pepper

1. Combine the couscous and boiling water in a small bowl. Stir once, then cover with a plate or pot lid. Let sit for 5 minutes, then fluff gently with a fork.

2. In a large bowl, combine the parsley, mint, tomatoes, scallions, and couscous. Add the olive oil, lemon zest and juice, salt. and pepper, and toss well. You can eat it right away, but the longer it sits, the better it will be.

INGREDIENT TIP: Couscous is made with wheat flour, like pasta, so look for whole-wheat couscous. Bulgur is cracked, parboiled wheat, so it is more of a whole, intact grain.

PER SERVING: Calories: 169; Total Fat: 14g; Saturated Fat: 2g; Cholesterol: 0mg; Sodium: 185mg; Carbohydrates: 10g; Fiber: 4g; Added Sugars: 0g; Protein: 3g; Potassium: 530mg; Vitamin K: 1,023mcg

MIDDLE EASTERN BULGUR PILAF

DASH • MEDITERRANEAN • VEGETARIAN • PORTABLE

Pilaf is a Middle Eastern or Indian dish of rice or wheat cooked in stock with meat and/or vegetables. In this case we're using bulgur, precooked cracked wheat. It's a whole grain that cooks quickly and can be used in place of rice or quinoa. Add spinach, chopped tomatoes, or chopped carrots for more vegetables. Add walnuts for a heartier vegetarian dish, or Pan-Seared Chicken (page 120) for a meaty meal. Of course, you can use fresh bell peppers and onions if you like, but they will take a few more minutes to cook.

Serves 4

Hands-on time: 15 min

Total time: 30 min

2 tablespoons extra-virgin olive oil, divided

2 cups frozen sliced red bell peppers and onions

2 garlic cloves, minced

1 cup uncooked bulgur

½ cup sliced sun-dried tomatoes in oil

2¼ cups reduced-sodium vegetable broth

8 ounces fresh snap peas

2 tablespoons red wine vinegar

¼ teaspoon freshly ground black pepper

⅓ cup crumbled feta cheese

1. Heat 1 tablespoon of oil in a large skillet over medium-high heat. When it is hot, add the peppers and onions. Cook, stirring occasionally, until the vegetables are thawed, then turn the heat down to medium and add the garlic.

2. Stir for about a minute, then add the bulgur, sun-dried tomatoes, and broth. Turn the heat back up to bring it to a boil, then turn it down again, cover, and simmer for 12 minutes (set a timer).

3. Meanwhile, trim and cut the snap peas into bite-size pieces. When the timer goes off, add them to the bulgur, then set the timer for another 5 minutes.

4. When the timer goes off again, stir in the red wine vinegar, black pepper, and remaining 1 tablespoon of olive oil. Top with the feta cheese.

FLAVOR BOOST: Top with fresh parsley, cilantro, or mint if you like.

PER SERVING: Calories: 300; Total Fat: 12g; Saturated Fat: 3g; Cholesterol: 11mg; Sodium: 246mg; Carbohydrates: 41g; Fiber: 8g; Added Sugars: 0g; Protein: 10g; Potassium: 528mg; Vitamin K: 5mcg

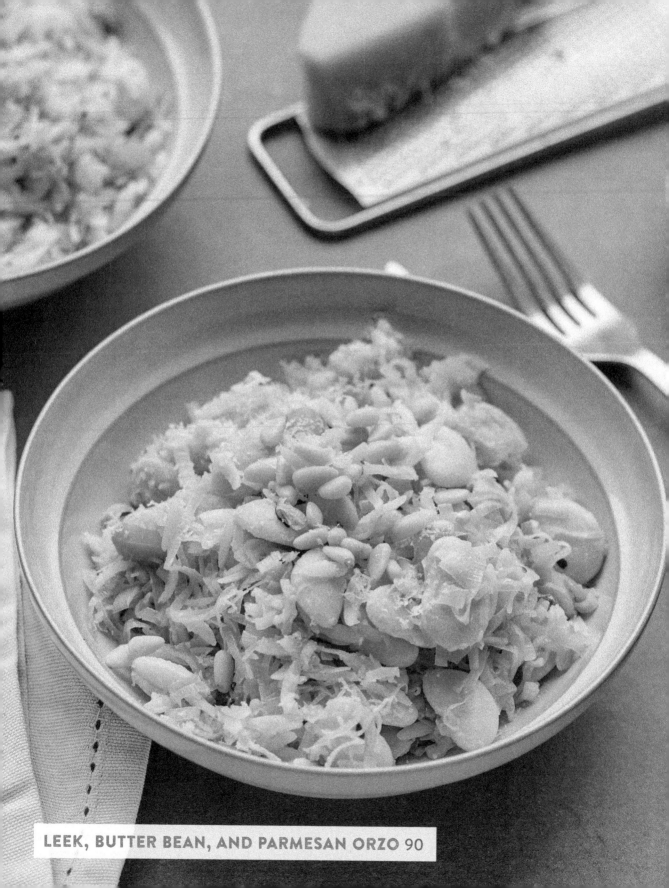

LEEK, BUTTER BEAN, AND PARMESAN ORZO 90

CHAPTER FOUR

VEGETARIAN AND VEGAN ENTRÉES

PILE-IT-HIGH VEGGIE SANDWICH

DASH • MEDITERRANEAN • VEGAN • NO-COOK • PORTABLE

It's a salad in a sandwich—and also a great way to use up leftover cooked vegetables! This is the perfect meal for a hot day, or as a side to go with a bowl of soup or chili. You can use the filling in wraps, too. If you don't have avocado, substitute a slice of cheese (unless you need the meal to be vegan).

Serves 2

Hands-on time: 15 min

Total time: 15 min

2 teaspoons red wine vinegar

1 teaspoon extra-virgin olive oil

¼ teaspoon ground cumin

⅓ cup shredded carrot (about 1 carrot)

2 tablespoons hummus, divided

4 slices whole-grain multigrain bread

½ avocado, sliced

6 (½-inch-thick) slices Simple Roasted Peppers (page 61) or jarred roasted red peppers, drained well

4 green lettuce leaves

1. In a small bowl, whisk together the vinegar, oil, and cumin. Add the carrot and toss well, then set aside to marinate for 10 minutes.

2. Spread 1 tablespoon of hummus on each of two slices of bread.

3. Divide the avocado slices between the other two pieces of bread. Top with the roasted peppers and lettuce.

4. Drain the carrots, and add them on top of the lettuce. Close the sandwiches and enjoy.

FLAVOR BOOST: Add freshly ground black pepper or red pepper flakes to the oil and vinegar before marinating the carrots.

PER SERVING: Calories: 384; Total Fat: 16g; Saturated Fat: 2g; Cholesterol: 0mg; Sodium: 463mg; Carbohydrates: 48g; Fiber: 11g; Added Sugars: 0g; Protein: 14g; Potassium: 619mg; Vitamin K: 30mcg

SPROUTED-GRAIN PIZZA TOAST

MEDITERRANEAN • VEGETARIAN • ONE POT

To make a heart-healthier pizza, start with a whole-grain crust. Sprouted-grain toast makes for a quick and nutritious pizza base. Use the toppings suggested here, or try arugula sautéed briefly in olive oil, oil-packed sun-dried tomatoes, roasted red peppers, sliced olives, cooked chicken, goat cheese, and/or grated Parmesan cheese. This is a fun meal to do with a group; put out the toppings and let everyone make their own. Pair the pizzas with a light salad or crunchy raw vegetables for a balanced meal.

Serves 2

Hands-on time: 22 min

Total time: 30 min

1 tablespoon canola or sunflower oil

4 slices sprouted-grain bread

2 tablespoons extra-virgin olive oil

½ teaspoon stir-in garlic paste

½ cup shredded mozzarella cheese

½ cup cherry tomatoes, thinly sliced, divided

¼ cup fresh basil leaves, stacked, rolled, and thinly sliced, divided

1. Preheat the oven to 400°F.

2. Brush a thin layer of canola or sunflower oil on a baking sheet. Spread out the bread on the sheet. Toast in the oven for 2½ minutes, flip the bread over and toast for 2½ minutes more.

3. Meanwhile, mix the olive oil and garlic paste in a small bowl.

4. Remove the toast from the oven, and brush some garlic oil on each slice. Add some mozzarella to each slice. Top each with half of the cherry tomatoes and basil.

5. Toast for another 5 minutes, until the cheese is melted and the crust is just starting to brown.

INGREDIENT TIP: If you don't have stir-in garlic paste, make your own with ¼ teaspoon each minced garlic and extra-virgin olive oil.

LEFTOVERS: You're not likely to have leftovers, but if you do, reheat them in a 300°F oven for a few minutes.

PER SERVING: Calories: 480; Total Fat: 28g; Saturated Fat: 6g; Cholesterol: 18mg; Sodium: 548mg; Carbohydrates: 41g; Fiber: 8g; Added Sugars: 0g; Protein: 17g; Potassium: 369mg; Vitamin K: 29mcg

SWEET SPOT LENTIL SALAD

DASH • MEDITERRANEAN • VEGETARIAN • NO COOK • PORTABLE

This colorful, crunchy salad is right in the heart-healthy sweet spot: satisfying, quick, and nutritious. Lentils are rich in protein and iron, making them a great alternative to meat, and they're also affordable, convenient, and high in fiber and blood pressure–friendly potassium. If you don't have these exact vegetables, substitute others—just look for a variety of colors.

Serves 3

Hands-on time: 20 min

Total time: 20 min

For the dressing

3 tablespoons apple cider vinegar

2 tablespoons extra-virgin olive oil

1 teaspoon water

1 teaspoon Dijon mustard

¼ teaspoon salt

¼ teaspoon freshly ground black pepper

For the salad

1 (15-ounce) can lentils, rinsed and drained

1 red bell pepper, seeded and chopped

½ cup frozen corn kernels, thawed

½ cup chopped snap peas

½ cup diced Jarlsberg cheese

¼ cup chopped fresh cilantro

1. In a large bowl, whisk together the vinegar, oil, water, mustard, salt, and pepper.

2. Add the lentils, bell pepper, corn, snap peas, cheese, and cilantro, and toss with the dressing.

LEFTOVERS: Make this dish on Sunday and you'll have a ready-to-go, heart-healthy lunch for the next few days. Store in an airtight container in the refrigerator and eat chilled or at room temperature.

PER SERVING: Calories: 440; Total Fat: 17g; Saturated Fat: 5g; Cholesterol: 20mg; Sodium: 422mg; Carbohydrates: 50g; Fiber: 17g; Added Sugars: 0g; Protein: 25g; Potassium: 893mg; Vitamin K: 15mcg

BLACK BEAN POTLUCK SALAD

DASH • MEDITERRANEAN • VEGETARIAN • PORTABLE

The bright, contrasting colors in this salad make it a perfect choice for a potluck lunch or dinner. It's a flavorful crowd pleaser, and you'll be sure to have a light, nutritious option on the communal table. For more color and nutrition, add avocado, chopped jalapeño peppers, or more chopped bell peppers in a variety of colors.

Serves 4

Hands-on time: 25 min

Total time: 30 min

For the salad

¾ cup uncooked quinoa

1 (15-ounce) can no-salt-added black beans, rinsed and drained

1 large tomato, chopped

½ red bell pepper, chopped

½ cup chopped red onion

1 cup frozen corn kernels (they will thaw by the time the salad is ready)

1 cup chopped fresh cilantro

⅔ cup crumbled or cubed feta cheese

For the dressing

3 tablespoons extra-virgin olive oil

2 tablespoons red wine vinegar

2 garlic cloves, minced

2 teaspoons chili powder

¼ teaspoon table salt

1. Start the quinoa cooking according to the package directions.

2. Meanwhile, make the dressing: In a large bowl, whisk together the olive oil, vinegar, garlic, chili powder, and salt.

3. Add the black beans, tomato, bell pepper, onion, corn, and cilantro to the bowl with the dressing, and toss to coat well.

4. When the quinoa is cooked, add it to the salad and toss well. Top with the feta cheese. Serve right away or cover and refrigerate—it gets better with time.

SUBSTITUTION TIP: Make this salad vegan by leaving out the feta cheese and sprinkling on some toasted pumpkin seeds.

PER SERVING: Calories: 423; Total Fat: 19g; Saturated Fat: 5g; Cholesterol: 22mg; Sodium: 372mg; Carbohydrates: 49g; Fiber: 10g; Added Sugars: 0g; Protein: 16g; Potassium: 704mg; Vitamin K: 23mcg

SWISS CHARD, BLACKBERRY, AND QUINOA SALAD

DASH • MEDITERRANEAN • VEGETARIAN • PORTABLE

Swiss chard, like most leafy greens, is packed with nutrients, and it makes for a fresh, hearty salad. Like kale, chard is best sliced into very thin ribbons and dressed well for a salad. The stems are edible and crunchy—just trim and chop them into bite-size pieces, as you would with celery. Then stack the chard leaves and roll them tightly. Cut the roll into ¼-inch slices, giving you long chard ribbons. Another bonus: This salad won't be wilted and soggy the next day! Add the pumpkin seeds right before serving so they stay crisp.

Serves 4

Hands-on time: 30 min

Total time: 30 min

For the salad

¾ cup uncooked quinoa

½ cup salted shelled pumpkin seeds

1 bunch Swiss chard

1 cup blackberries

1 cup canned lentils, rinsed and drained

⅓ cup crumbled goat cheese

For the dressing

3 tablespoons extra-virgin olive oil

3 tablespoons freshly squeezed lemon juice (about 1 lemon)

2 teaspoons honey

¼ teaspoon salt

¼ teaspoon freshly ground black pepper

1. Start the quinoa cooking according to the package directions. Put an empty bowl in the freezer to chill.

2. While the quinoa is cooking, toast the pumpkin seeds in a small, dry skillet for 3 to 4 minutes, watching closely so you don't burn them. Remove from the heat and slide them onto a plate as soon as they start to brown.

3. Trim the chard stems. Stack the leaves, and slice thinly.

4. Whisk together the olive oil, lemon juice, honey, salt, and pepper in a small bowl.

5. When the quinoa is done, transfer it to the chilled bowl and let it cool on the countertop for 5 minutes. Add the chard to the quinoa, then add the dressing and toss to coat thoroughly.

6. Add the blackberries, lentils, goat cheese, and toasted pumpkin seeds. Gently toss.

SUBSTITUTION TIP: This salad also goes nicely with grilled chicken or steak. You can leave out the lentils and cut the amount of goat cheese and pumpkin seeds in half.

PER SERVING: Calories: 427; Total Fat: 23g; Saturated Fat: 5g; Cholesterol: 9mg; Sodium: 444mg; Carbohydrates: 41g; Fiber: 10g; Added Sugars: 3g; Protein: 17g; Potassium: 757mg; Vitamin K: 463mcg

SWEET EDAMAME AND QUINOA

DASH • MEDITERRANEAN • VEGAN • PORTABLE

This salad can be a satisfying meatless meal, or you can cut the portions in half for a satisfying side salad. Edamame are whole soybeans—kind of a cross between peas and lima beans. You can buy them in their pods or shelled (more convenient!) in the freezer section of the supermarket. Look for shredded carrots in the produce section (you'll need about ½ cup), or toss a carrot in the food processor, if that's easier than grating it by hand.

Serves 3

Hands-on time: 20 min

Total time: 20 min

For the salad

½ cup uncooked quinoa

1 (5-ounce) package baby kale

1 medium carrot, peeled and grated

1 (11-ounce) can no-sugar-added mandarin orange segments, drained

1 cup frozen shelled edamame, thawed

⅓ cup slivered almonds

For the dressing

2 tablespoons canola or sunflower oil

2 tablespoons rice vinegar

1½ tablespoons reduced-sodium soy sauce

1 teaspoon minced fresh ginger

1. Start the quinoa cooking according to the package directions.

2. Meanwhile, make the dressing: Whisk together the oil, vinegar, soy sauce, and ginger in a large bowl.

3. Remove any long, tough stems from the kale. Then combine the kale, carrot, and mandarins in a large salad bowl.

4. When the quinoa is done, add the edamame to the pot and cover. Set aside, off the heat, for 5 minutes to steam.

5. Add the quinoa, edamame, and dressing to the salad bowl and toss. Top with the almonds. Serve warm or chilled.

COOKING TIP: Ginger is a great way to add flavor to lower-sodium food. To make it easier to use, chop up a big piece all at once, by hand or in a mini-chopper. Freeze it flat in a freezer bag, and just break off a chunk when you need it.

PER SERVING: Calories: 368; Total Fat: 19g; Saturated Fat: 1g; Cholesterol: 0mg; Sodium: 379mg; Carbohydrates: 40g; Fiber: 9g; Added Sugars: 0g; Protein: 14g; Potassium: 893mg; Vitamin K: 355mcg

CHICKPEAS, TOMATOES, AND SWISS CHARD

DASH • MEDITERRANEAN • VEGAN • ONE POT

If you have a backyard garden, try growing chard. It's tolerant of both warm and cool temperatures, but it does need plenty of water. Any color of chard will be packed with vitamins A, C, and K, potassium, and calcium, but this salad looks best with rainbow or red chard. Served over brown rice or another grain, this makes a quick, light meal.

Serves 4

Hands-on time: 20 min

Total time: 20 min

1 bunch Swiss chard

2 tablespoons extra-virgin olive oil

1 onion, thinly sliced

2 garlic cloves, minced

1 teaspoon ground cumin

½ teaspoon red pepper flakes

1 (14-ounce) can diced tomatoes seasoned with basil and garlic

1 (15-ounce) can no-salt-added chickpeas, rinsed and drained

Zest and juice of 1 lemon (about 3 tablespoons juice)

½ cup chopped walnuts

Freshly ground black pepper

1. Trim the chard, then chop the stems and leaves; keep the stems and leaves separate.

2. Heat the oil in a large skillet over medium heat. When it is hot, add the onion and garlic and cook, stirring occasionally, for 3 to 4 minutes.

3. Add the chard stems and continue to cook until the onion is softened, 3 to 4 minutes more.

4. Add the cumin and red pepper flakes, and cook for 1 minute. Add the tomatoes with their juice and the chickpeas, and cook until warm, 3 to 4 minutes.

5. Add the chard leaves, cover, and cook until wilted, about 2 minutes.

6. Remove from the heat, and add the lemon zest and juice, walnuts, and pepper.

INGREDIENT TIP: Out-of-season tomatoes have almost no flavor, which is why I use canned tomatoes here. But if you can get ripe, fresh tomatoes in season, chop up 3 or 4 of them instead. Add a little dried basil and up to ¼ teaspoon salt.

PER SERVING: Calories: 317; Total Fat: 18g; Saturated Fat: 2g; Cholesterol: 0mg; Sodium: 482mg; Carbohydrates: 31g; Fiber: 9g; Added Sugars: 0g; Protein: 11g; Potassium: 922mg; Vitamin K: 949mcg

CHICKPEA-ALMOND CURRY

DASH • MEDITERRANEAN • VEGAN • ONE POT

Curry paste or powder is a mixture of spices that vary from region to region in India. Curry paste is typically spicier than the powder and includes fresh ingredients such as garlic and ginger in oil, in addition to the spices. Red curry is usually hotter than green. Either way, cook it for a minute after adding it to the pan to bring out the flavors. Use more for a spicier dish, and substitute curry powder if you prefer it mild—start with ½ teaspoon. This dish works well with frozen stir-fry vegetables, or you can chop fresh ones if you have them. You can also use cashew or peanut butter instead of almond butter. Serve over brown rice, farro, or quinoa.

Serves 4

Hands-on time: 30 min

Total time: 30 min

1 tablespoon canola or sunflower oil

1 onion, chopped

2 cups stir-fry vegetables, fresh or frozen

1 tablespoon grated fresh ginger

2 teaspoons red or green curry paste

1 teaspoon ground turmeric

1 (14-ounce) can diced no-salt-added tomatoes

1 (15-ounce) can no-salt-added-chickpeas, rinsed and drained

¼ cup smooth almond butter

2 cups reduced-sodium vegetable broth

1. Heat the oil in a large skillet over medium-high heat. When it is hot, add the onion and cook until translucent, 4 to 5 minutes. Add the stir-fry vegetables, and cook for 3 to 4 minutes. Add the ginger, curry paste, and turmeric, and cook for 1 more minute.

2. Stir in the tomatoes with their juice, chickpeas, almond butter, and broth, and bring to a boil. Turn the heat down to low and simmer, stirring occasionally, for 5 to 10 minutes, until warmed through.

FLAVOR BOOST: For a twist, add a squeeze of lime juice. Garnish each serving with a few slivered almonds.

PER SERVING: Calories: 308; Total Fat: 14g; Saturated Fat: 1g; Cholesterol: 0mg; Sodium: 348mg; Carbohydrates: 34g; Fiber: 10g; Added Sugars: 0g; Protein: 12g; Potassium: 769mg; Vitamin K: 10mcg

BLACK BEAN QUESADILLAS

DASH • MEDITERRANEAN • VEGETARIAN • PORTABLE

This is a quick crowd-pleaser you can pull together from pantry staples (substitute ½ cup frozen corn if you don't have a bell pepper on hand). Between the beans and the whole-wheat tortillas, it's high in fiber, too, which can help keep both your heart and your gut healthy. Be sure to look for lower-sodium salsa and tortilla brands. Serve with crunchy raw vegetables or a light salad. Dip in some extra salsa, plain Greek yogurt, or sour cream if you like.

Serves 4

Hands-on time: 25 min

Total time: 25 min

1 (15-ounce) can no-salt-added black beans, rinsed and drained

¼ cup Fresh Tomato Salsa (page 182) or lower-sodium store-bought salsa

¾ cup shredded Cheddar cheese, divided

1 red bell pepper, seeded and chopped, divided

2 tablespoons canola or sunflower oil, divided

4 large, whole-grain tortillas

1. Blend the beans and salsa together in a food processor. If you don't have a food processor, mash them in a large bowl with a fork or a potato masher.

2. Spread one-fourth of the bean mixture (about ½ cup) on each tortilla. Sprinkle each with 3 tablespoons of cheese and one-fourth of the bell pepper (about ¼ cup). Fold in half.

3. Preheat a large, heavy skillet over medium heat. Add 1 tablespoon of oil to the skillet and spread it around. Place the first two quesadillas in the skillet. Cover and cook until the quesadillas are crispy on the bottom, about 2 minutes. Flip and cook until crispy on the other side, about 2 minutes more.

4. Use the remaining 1 tablespoon of oil to cook the remaining two quesadillas, keeping the first two warm in the oven if needed.

FLAVOR BOOST: If you like heat, add chopped jalapeño pepper or a dash of hot sauce to the black bean mixture in step 1.

PER SERVING: Calories: 438; Total Fat: 21g; Saturated Fat: 5g; Cholesterol: 21mg; Sodium: 561mg; Carbohydrates: 46g; Fiber: 12g; Added Sugars: 0g; Protein: 17g; Potassium: 511mg; Vitamin K: 12mcg

PANTRY BEANS AND RICE

DASH • MEDITERRANEAN • VEGETARIAN

You can stock the ingredients for this dish in your pantry, fridge, and freezer so they're ready to pull out when you have no time for a grocery run. The recipe is also extremely flexible, so you can use whatever you have on hand—substitute another green vegetable if you don't have broccoli, and chop up a small fresh onion if you don't have frozen onions. To make this dish vegan, substitute ½ cup toasted shelled pumpkin seeds for the cheese.

Serves 3

Hands-on time: 25 min

Total time: 25 min

¾ cup uncooked parboiled brown rice

2 teaspoons extra-virgin olive oil

1 cup fresh or frozen chopped onion

1 (15-ounce) can no-salt-added pinto beans, rinsed and drained

1 (14-ounce) can no-salt-added diced tomatoes

⅔ cup spicy salsa

1 cup frozen broccoli florets

1 tablespoon freshly squeezed lime juice

⅔ cup shredded aged Cheddar cheese

½ teaspoon red pepper flakes (optional)

1. Cook the rice according to the package directions.

2. In a large skillet, heat the oil over medium-high heat. Add the onion and cook until soft, 4 to 5 minutes. Then add the beans, tomatoes with their juice, and salsa. Bring to a boil.

3. Add the broccoli, and when the liquid returns to a boil, turn the heat to low and simmer for 2 to 3 minutes. Remove from the heat when the broccoli is crisp-tender but still bright green.

4. Add the rice when it's done cooking. Stir in the lime juice, and top with the shredded Cheddar and red pepper flakes (if using).

LEFTOVERS: Whenever you cook brown rice or barley, make a big batch and freeze it in smaller containers. Reheat in the microwave with a tablespoon of water for a minute or two, depending on the quantity.

PER SERVING: Calories: 479; Total Fat: 14g; Saturated Fat: 5g; Cholesterol: 25mg; Sodium: 442mg; Carbohydrates: 72g; Fiber: 13g; Added Sugars: 0g; Protein: 20g; Potassium: 1,050mg; Vitamin K: 49mcg

POLENTA WITH TOMATOES AND BLACK BEANS

DASH · MEDITERRANEAN · VEGETARIAN

Quick-cooking cornmeal is a light, creamy indulgence, and the beans and vegetables in this dish provide plenty of fiber and other nutrients normally contributed by whole grains.

Serves 3

Hands-on time: 25 min

Total time: 25 min

1 tablespoon extra-virgin olive oil

1 small yellow onion, chopped

2 garlic cloves, minced

1 teaspoon dried thyme

1 (15-ounce) can no-salt-added black beans, rinsed and drained

1 (14-ounce) can no-salt-added diced tomatoes

⅔ cup cornmeal (also called corn grits)

2⅔ cups water, divided

1 bunch spinach, large stems removed

½ cup grated Parmesan cheese

1. Heat the oil in a large sauté pan over medium heat. Sauté the onion, garlic, and thyme until the onion is soft, 3 to 5 minutes. Add the beans and the tomatoes with their juice, and simmer over a low heat while you cook the polenta.

2. Combine the cornmeal with ⅔ cup of water in a small bowl. Set aside.

3. In a small saucepan, bring the remaining 2 cups of water to a boil over high heat. Reduce the heat to low, and stir in the cornmeal-water mixture. Stir frequently until the polenta is smooth and creamy, about 10 minutes, adding more water if needed.

4. When the polenta is ready, stir the spinach into the beans and tomatoes, cover, and cook until the spinach is wilted, about 2 minutes. Stir to incorporate.

5. Spoon the polenta into bowls, and top with the beans, tomatoes, and spinach. Sprinkle with the Parmesan.

COOKING TIP: Use a 5-ounce bag of prewashed spinach, frozen onion, and garlic stir-in paste if you want to shave a few minutes off of this already-quick weeknight meal.

PER SERVING: Calories: 387; Total Fat: 10g; Saturated Fat: 3g; Cholesterol: 9mg; Sodium: 263mg; Carbohydrates: 57g; Fiber: 11g; Added Sugars: 0g; Protein: 18g; Potassium: 929mg; Vitamin K: 241mcg

CRUNCHY PEANUT FRIED RICE

DASH • MEDITERRANEAN • VEGETARIAN • ONE POT

This updated version of the takeout classic has more veggies and protein and less sodium, and it's faster than delivery. A 2015 study showed that people who regularly ate peanuts were substantially less likely to have died of any cause—particularly heart disease—over the study period than those who rarely ate nuts, echoing findings from earlier studies.

A bag of fresh coleslaw mix (typically chopped cabbage, carrots, and other veggies) makes this dish come together super quick; choose the most colorful one you can find. If you don't have peanut oil, just use a neutral oil like canola. You can substitute egg whites, but include at least one yolk for the flavor, nutrition, and color.

Serves 4

Hands-on time: 20 min

Total time: 25 min

2 tablespoons reduced-sodium soy sauce

3 tablespoons rice vinegar

1 tablespoon sugar

5 large eggs

2 tablespoons peanut oil

3 cups cooked brown rice

½ cup frozen peas

1 (14-ounce) bag coleslaw mix

1 teaspoon minced fresh ginger

3 garlic cloves, chopped

½ cup roughly chopped lightly salted peanuts

1. Mix the soy sauce, vinegar, and sugar in a small bowl. Set aside.

2. Crack the eggs into a bowl, and beat gently.

3. Heat the oil in a large skillet over high heat. When it is hot, add the rice and stir-fry for 2 minutes. Add the peas and coleslaw mix, and cook for 3 minutes. Add the ginger, and garlic and cook for 1 more minute.

4. Turn the heat down to medium. Push the vegetables and rice to the side, and add the eggs. Stir until lightly scrambled.

5. Pour the sauce over the rice and eggs, and mix well. Top with the peanuts.

FLAVOR BOOST TIP: Add a sprinkle of red pepper flakes, a squeeze of lime, or chopped fresh cilantro.

PER SERVING: Calories: 508; Total Fat: 24g; Saturated Fat: 5g; Cholesterol: 233mg; Sodium: 494mg; Carbohydrates: 56g; Fiber: 7g; Added Sugars: 3g; Protein: 20g; Potassium: 401mg; Vitamin K: 18mcg

FARRO AND VEGETABLE RAINBOW BOWL

DASH • MEDITERRANEAN • VEGAN • PORTABLE

For this creative do-it-yourself dinner, you can either toss everything together or put out each ingredient and let everyone make their own bowl. Leave out the butternut squash if time is tight or you can't find it precut. Use what you have: avocado, shredded carrots, tomatoes, hemp seeds, pumpkin seeds, snap peas, and anything else.

Serves 4

Hands-on time: 30 min

Total time: 30 min

1 (12-ounce) package fresh or frozen cubed butternut squash

1 tablespoon canola or sunflower oil

⅛ teaspoon salt

½ cup uncooked farro

4 cups mixed greens, torn into bite-size pieces

1 red, yellow, or orange bell pepper, seeded and chopped

¾ cup hummus

1 (15-ounce) can no-salt-added chickpeas, rinsed and drained

½ cup sunflower seeds

½ cup pickled beets, chopped

1. Preheat the oven to 420°F. Line a rimmed baking sheet with parchment paper. Put a large salad bowl in the freezer.

2. In a large bowl, toss the squash with the oil, and sprinkle with the salt. Spread out the squash on the baking sheet. Roast for 18 to 25 minutes, until the squash is tender, tossing every 10 minutes so it doesn't burn. (Fresh takes longer than frozen.)

3. Meanwhile, cook the farro according to the package directions.

4. When the farro is done, transfer it to the chilled bowl and let it cool on the countertop for 5 minutes. Add the greens, bell pepper, hummus, chickpeas, and sunflower seeds to the farro, and toss well.

5. Top with the beets and roasted squash.

INGREDIENT TIP: Farro is a whole grain derived from wheat. It's one of the oldest cultivated grains in the world. Farro grains look a bit like brown rice, but are chewier and have a rich, nutty flavor. Most supermarkets carry it, but use quinoa if you can't find it.

PER SERVING: Calories: 408; Total Fat: 13g; Saturated Fat: 1g; Cholesterol: 0mg; Sodium: 399mg; Carbohydrates: 60g; Fiber: 12g; Added Sugars: 0g; Protein: 16g; Potassium: 695mg; Vitamin K: 73mcg

LEEK, BUTTER BEAN, AND PARMESAN ORZO

DASH • MEDITERRANEAN • VEGETARIAN

This dish is proof that vegetables and beans can be comfort food. Orzo is a small, short pasta that looks like grains of rice, and it cooks very quickly. If you can't find it, try angel hair pasta, which you break in half before cooking.

Serves 4

Hands-on time: 25 min

Total time: 30 min

2 tablespoons extra-virgin olive oil

1 garlic clove, minced

1 pound leeks (white and very light green parts only), thinly sliced

½ red bell pepper

¾ cup uncooked orzo

Zest and juice of 1 lemon (about 3 tablespoons juice)

1 (15-ouce) can butter beans, rinsed and drained

2 tablespoons fresh thyme leaves or 1 teaspoon dried

½ cup grated Parmesan cheese

¼ cup pine nuts

1. Heat the olive oil in a large, nonstick skillet over medium heat. When it's hot, add the garlic and stir for 30 seconds or so. Stir in the sliced leeks. Cover and cook, stirring occasionally, until soft, 8 to 10 minutes. Add a splash of water if it gets dry.

2. While the leeks are cooking, seed and dice the bell pepper and add it to the skillet.

3. Meanwhile, in another pot, cook the orzo just to al dente, according to the package directions. Scoop out ¼ cup of the pasta cooking water before draining.

4. When the leeks are soft, stir in the cooked orzo, reserved ¼ cup of cooking water, and the lemon zest and juice. Add the beans, cover, and cook to warm them, about 2 minutes.

5. Remove from the heat, and gently stir in the cheese. Top with the pine nuts.

INGREDIENT TIP: Butter beans are also known as lima beans. If you can't find them, substitute any other white bean.

PER SERVING: Calories: 451; Total Fat: 17g; Saturated Fat: 3g; Cholesterol: 7mg; Sodium: 324mg; Carbohydrates: 60g; Fiber: 11g; Added Sugars: 0g; Protein: 17g; Potassium: 578mg; Vitamin K: 51mcg

PASTA WITH GREENS AND BEANS

DASH • MEDITERRANEAN • VEGETARIAN

In this hearty dish, linguine is covered in a deliciously creamy sauce, with heart-healthy fats from walnuts. You'll get plenty of fiber and other nutrients from the beans and chard.

Serves 5

Hands-on time: 30 min

Total time: 30 min

For the pasta

½ teaspoon salt

8 ounces uncooked linguine

1 tablespoon extra-virgin olive oil

2 garlic cloves, minced

1 bunch Swiss chard, trimmed, stems chopped, leaves sliced into thin ribbons

1 (15-ounce) can no-salt-added white beans, rinsed and drained

Zest and juice of 1 lemon (about 3 tablespoons juice)

¼ cup grated Parmesan cheese

Freshly ground black pepper

For the sauce

1 cup part-skim ricotta cheese

¾ cup chopped walnuts

¼ cup grated Parmesan cheese

1 garlic clove, peeled

1. Fill a large pot with water, add the salt, and bring it to a boil over high heat. Cook the linguine to al dente, according to the package directions. Scoop out ½ cup of the pasta cooking water, then drain the pasta and leave it in the colander.

2. Return the pot to the stovetop over medium heat. Add the olive oil, garlic, and chard stems. Sauté for 2 to 3 minutes, then add the chard leaves. Cook just until wilted, about 2 minutes.

3. To make the sauce, blend the ricotta cheese, walnuts, Parmesan cheese, and garlic in a food processor or blender. Slowly add the reserved ½ cup of cooking water to thin the sauce.

→

4. Return the pasta to the pot, along with the sauce and white beans. Toss well and heat through.

5. Add the lemon zest and juice. Serve topped with the Parmesan cheese and pepper.

PER SERVING: Calories: 495; Total Fat: 22g; Saturated Fat: 5g; Cholesterol: 21mg; Sodium: 440mg; Carbohydrates: 55g; Fiber: 7g; Added Sugars: 0g; Protein: 23g; Potassium: 775mg; Vitamin K: 756mcg

BROCCOLI AND PASTA WITH PEANUT SAUCE

DASH • MEDITERRANEAN • VEGAN

If you aren't a broccoli fan, think of this as pasta with peanut sauce hiding a little broccoli. It's a weeknight staple in our house, and everyone gobbles it up. You can find ready-to-cook broccoli florets in the produce section, if you're short on time. Or use frozen broccoli—it cooks a bit faster, so add it just 2 minutes before the pasta is done. Add Crispy Tofu (page 186) or Pan-Seared Chicken (page 120) if you want more protein.

Serves 4

Hands-on time: 25 min

Total time: 25 min

8 ounces uncooked whole-wheat rotini

1 pint cherry tomatoes

⅔ cup reduced-sodium vegetable broth

½ cup natural peanut butter

3 tablespoons rice vinegar

1 tablespoon canola or sunflower oil

1 teaspoon toasted sesame oil

1½ teaspoons reduced-sodium soy sauce

1 garlic clove, chopped

3½ cups broccoli florets (about 1 pound)

1. Bring a large pot of water to a boil over high heat. Cook the rotini to al dente, according to the package directions.

2. While the pasta is cooking, combine the tomatoes, broth, peanut butter, vinegar, canola oil, sesame oil, soy sauce, and garlic in a medium pot over medium heat. Cook, stirring occasionally, until the tomatoes burst.

3. A few minutes before the pasta is finished cooking, add the broccoli to the pasta pot. When it starts boiling again, turn it back down and simmer for another 3 minutes. Drain and return the pasta and broccoli to the pasta pot.

4. Add the sauce, and toss to coat.

FLAVOR BOOST: Sprinkle on some red pepper flakes if you like heat.

PER SERVING: Calories: 490; Total Fat: 23g; Saturated Fat: 3g; Cholesterol: 0mg; Sodium: 210mg; Carbohydrates: 55g; Fiber: 10g; Added Sugars: 0g; Protein: 18g; Potassium: 671mg; Vitamin K: 11mcg

NATURE'S VEGGIE BURGER

DASH • MEDITERRANEAN • VEGETARIAN

The quest to eat more plants and less meat leads many people to veggie burgers. Unfortunately, most store-bought veggie burgers are high in sodium and have lengthy, intimidating ingredient lists. They can be complicated to make from scratch, too. Portobello mushrooms are a simple solution: meaty, rich in umami flavor, and wonderful grilled and eaten like a hamburger. Look for the biggest ones you can find, as they shrink when cooked.

Serves 4

Hands-on time: 15 min

Total time: 25 min

3 tablespoons extra-virgin olive oil

1 tablespoon chopped garlic

4 very large portobello mushrooms, gills and stems removed

4 crusty whole-grain rolls *or* 1 multigrain baguette cut into 3-inch-long pieces

½ cup crumbled goat cheese

Freshly ground black pepper (optional)

4 green lettuce leaves

1. Preheat a grill to medium. (Alternatively, preheat the oven to 425°F and line a rimmed baking sheet with aluminum foil.)

2. Mix the olive oil and the chopped garlic in a small bowl. Brush about half of the mixture on both sides of the mushrooms, and let them sit for 10 minutes.

3. Meanwhile, split open the rolls. Drizzle the remaining garlic-infused oil onto the bottom half of each roll, including the garlic if you like. Spread about 2 tablespoons of goat cheese on the top half of each roll.

4. Place the mushrooms on the grill, cap-side down, close the lid, and grill until they're brown and tender, 5 to 10 minutes, turning once. (Or place them on the foil-lined sheet, cap-side down, and roast in the oven for 12 minutes on each side.)

5. Put one mushroom on the bottom of each roll. Add a grind of pepper, if desired. Top with a leaf of lettuce and then the top of the roll.

SUBSTITUTION TIP: Swap the cheese for avocado for a vegan alternative. Or have them both!

COOKING TIP: Use a spoon to easily remove the gills from portobello mushrooms.

PER SERVING: Calories: 307; Total Fat: 17g; Saturated Fat: 5g; Cholesterol: 14mg; Sodium: 276mg; Carbohydrates: 26g; Fiber: 4g; Added Sugars: 0g; Protein: 6g; Potassium: 338mg; Vitamin K: 13mcg

LEMON-TAHINI AND TOFU ENERGY BOWL

DASH • MEDITERRANEAN • VEGAN

Once you get this basic recipe down, feel free to experiment with different grains, vegetables, and proteins. Try chopped red cabbage, diced bell peppers, grated carrots, grated beets, baby spinach, arugula, avocado, slivered almonds, chicken, salmon...

Serves 4

Hands-on time: 30 min

Total time: 30 min

¾ cup uncooked quinoa

1 (12-ounce) package kale slaw (about 6 cups)

2 tablespoons extra-virgin olive oil

1 recipe Crispy Tofu (page 186)

1 recipe Lemon-Tahini Dressing (page 177)

2 tablespoons shelled pumpkin seeds

1. Cook the quinoa according to the package directions.

2. Pour the kale slaw into a medium bowl. Look for any pieces of kale wider than ¼ inch, and cut them into narrow ribbons. Drizzle the olive oil over the kale, and massage it into the leaves with your fingers to soften it.

3. Assemble the bowls: quinoa first, then the kale slaw, then the tofu. Drizzle each bowl with about 2 tablespoons of dressing, then top with the pumpkin seeds.

INGREDIENT TIP: Kale slaw conveniently combines chopped kale with other nutritious vegetables, including broccoli, cabbage, and carrots. If you can't find it, you can use broccoli slaw plus kale or a kale salad kit minus the dressing.

PER SERVING: Calories: 520; Total Fat: 34g; Saturated Fat: 4g; Cholesterol: 0mg; Sodium: 311mg; Carbohydrates: 37g; Fiber: 5g; Added Sugars: 0g; Protein: 18g; Potassium: 255mg; Vitamin K: 16mcg

SPICY WEEKNIGHT COCONUT TOFU CURRY

DASH • MEDITERRANEAN • VEGAN • ONE POT

Don't let the saturated fat in coconut milk scare you away from using it now and then. In moderation, in a home-cooked, plant-based meal like this, it's unlikely to make a difference. Curry paste is spicy, so use more or less of it, depending on your preference. Serve this dish over rice, farro, or quinoa.

Serves 4

Hands-on time: 20 min

Total time: 20 min

1½ pounds firm tofu

2 tablespoons canola or sunflower oil, divided

1 cup frozen diced onion

5 cups frozen stir-fry vegetables

1 tablespoon curry paste, plus more to taste

1 (14-ounce) can light coconut milk

1 teaspoon freshly squeezed lime juice

1 teaspoon reduced-sodium vegetable broth base or bouillon, if needed

1. Drain the tofu, and slice through its equator to make two flat blocks. Wrap them side by side in a couple of layers of clean kitchen or paper towel, and place a heavy book or frying pan on top. Let the tofu drain for at least 5 minutes. Cut the tofu slabs into 1-inch squares.

2. Heat 1 tablespoon of oil in a large skillet over medium-high heat. When it is shimmering, add the tofu. Let it cook undisturbed until golden brown on the bottom, about 5 minutes. Flip each piece, and cook until crispy on the other side, 4 to 5 minutes more. Transfer to a plate.

3. Add the remaining 1 tablespoon of oil to the skillet, then add the onion and stir-fry vegetables. Stir-fry for 2 minutes. Add the curry paste, and cook for another minute.

4. Add the coconut milk. When it starts to boil, reduce the heat to low and simmer for 5 minutes. Add the lime juice, and taste. If needed, add the vegetable base and/or more curry paste.

5. Return the tofu to the skillet, and stir to warm through.

PER SERVING: Calories: 367; Total Fat: 22g; Saturated Fat: 8g; Cholesterol: 0mg; Sodium: 486mg; Carbohydrates: 27g; Fiber: 8g; Added Sugars: 0g; Protein: 21g; Potassium: 677mg; Vitamin K: 51mcg

OPEN-FACED LEMON PEPPER TUNA MELT 100

CHAPTER FIVE

SEAFOOD ENTRÉES

OPEN-FACED LEMON PEPPER TUNA MELT

MEDITERRANEAN

The sodium in a tuna melt can be high. This version dials it back and uses lemon and pepper for flavor. Make it even easier by using a salt-free lemon pepper seasoning instead of the lemon juice, zest, and pepper. Substitute whole-wheat bread if you can't find sprouted grain. Pair with a simple salad like the Awesome Arugula Salad (page 56).

Serves 2

Hands-on time: 15 min

Total time: 15 min

2 teaspoons Better Butter (page 176) or nonhydrogenated margarine

2 slices sprouted-grain bread

1 (5-ounce) can sustainably sourced tuna, packed in water

2 teaspoons extra-virgin olive oil

2 teaspoons mayonnaise

1 teaspoon lemon zest

1 tablespoon freshly squeezed lemon juice

2 tablespoons finely chopped red onion (optional)

½ teaspoon red pepper flakes (optional)

Freshly ground black pepper

¼ cup shredded Cheddar cheese

1. Set the oven rack about 6 inches from the heat, and preheat the broiler.

2. Spread butter thinly on both sides of bread. Place the bread on a rimmed baking sheet. Toast the bread under the broiler until it is golden brown on both sides, about 2 minutes on each side. Watch it carefully to make sure it doesn't burn.

3. Drain the tuna well, and mash in a medium bowl with the oil, mayonnaise, lemon zest and juice, red onion and red pepper flakes (if using), and black pepper. Mix well.

4. Divide the tuna mixture between the two slices of bread, making sure the bread is completely covered. Sprinkle with the cheese.

5. Broil until the cheese is melted, 2 to 3 minutes.

INGREDIENT TIP: To find sustainably sourced fish, look for the Marine Stewardship Council (MSC) or Aquaculture Stewardship Council (ASC) logos. The Monterey Bay Aquarium's Seafood Watch app and website (www.seafoodwatch.org) can also guide you, as can a reputable fishmonger.

PER SERVING: Calories: 336; Total Fat: 19g; Saturated Fat: 5g; Cholesterol: 46mg; Sodium: 450mg; Carbohydrates: 21g; Fiber: 4g; Added Sugars: 0g; Protein: 22g; Potassium: 262mg; Vitamin K: 13mcg

TUNA, CASHEW, AND COUSCOUS SALAD

This salad works well with just about any intact whole grain: barley, bulgur, brown rice, wheat berries, and more. Broccoli slaw in available in the produce section, but if you can't find it, run some broccoli through the food processor using the grating disk. If you use tuna canned in water, mash it with 1 tablespoon of olive oil before mixing in all the other salad ingredients.

Serves 3

Hands-on time: 15 min

Total time: 15 min

½ cup uncooked whole-wheat couscous

¼ teaspoon salt

1 (5-ounce) can sustainably sourced tuna, packed in oil

1 bell pepper, any color, seeded and chopped

1 (12-ounce) package broccoli slaw (about 4 cups)

3 scallions, finely chopped

3 tablespoons red wine vinegar

2 tablespoons extra-virgin olive oil

1 teaspoon dried oregano

1 teaspoon dried thyme

½ teaspoon freshly ground black pepper

½ cup chopped unsalted roasted cashews

1. Prepare the couscous with the salt, according to the package directions. Transfer to a medium bowl, and let it cool until the other ingredients are ready.

2. Drain the tuna, and use a fork to mash it well in a large bowl. Add the bell pepper, broccoli slaw, scallions, vinegar, oil, oregano, thyme, and black pepper.

3. Add the couscous, and toss well. Adjust the seasonings, if desired. Top with the cashews.

INGREDIENT TIP: The sodium content of canned tuna varies greatly, so look for a lower-sodium brand (225mg or less per 2-ounce serving).

PER SERVING: Calories: 457; Total Fat: 24g; Saturated Fat: 4g; Cholesterol: 15mg; Sodium: 450mg; Carbohydrates: 39g; Fiber: 6g; Added Sugars: 0g; Protein: 24g; Potassium: 494mg; Vitamin K: 74mcg

SPICY SALMON SANDWICHES

DASH • MEDITERRANEAN • NO-COOK • PORTABLE

Canned salmon gives you the convenience of tuna, plus extra heart-healthy omega-3 fat. Surprisingly, most of the fat in mayonnaise is unsaturated too, so don't be afraid to add a little to moisten this up. For a lower-sodium option, replace the bread with a cooked grain and serve this dish as a salad.

Serves 4

Hands-on time: 15 min

Total time: 15 min

1 (6-ounce) can wild salmon, drained

2 tablespoons mayonnaise

¼ teaspoon Sriracha sauce

¼ teaspoon dried dill

½ cup shredded carrot

½ cup finely diced celery

½ cup canned, no-salt-added chickpeas, rinsed and drained

¼ cup unsalted sunflower seeds

8 slices sprouted-grain bread, toasted

4 lettuce leaves

1. In a medium bowl, mash the salmon together with the mayonnaise, Sriracha, and dill. Mix in the carrot, celery, chickpeas, and sunflower seeds.

2. Spread the salmon onto 4 slices of toast. Top with the lettuce and the other slices of toast.

INGREDIENT TIP: Sriracha is Thai hot sauce made from a paste of chiles, distilled vinegar, garlic, sugar, and salt. You can buy it at most grocery stores in the international aisle. It's quite spicy, so if you're not used to it, go easy! If you don't have any, you can use any hot sauce to spice up your salmon.

PER SERVING: Calories: 409; Total Fat: 14g; Saturated Fat: 2g; Cholesterol: 36mg; Sodium: 548mg; Carbohydrates: 47g; Fiber: 10g; Added Sugars: 0g; Protein: 24g; Potassium: 509mg; Vitamin K: 22mcg

ELECTRIC CHICKPEAS AND SHRIMP

This easy, no-cook dish makes an energizing light lunch when paired with a crusty whole-grain roll or toast. Or serve it without the shrimp as a zesty, fiber-boosting side dish. Add fresh avocado or serve it on a bed of lettuce, if you like.

Serves 3

Hands-on time: 20 min

Total time: 20 min

7 ounces sustainably sourced, frozen cooked shrimp, thawed and peeled

1 (15-ounce) can no-salt-added chickpeas, rinsed and drained

1 red bell pepper, seeded and diced

⅓ cup finely chopped red onion

1 garlic clove, finely chopped

½ cup red wine vinegar

3 tablespoons extra-virgin olive oil

½ teaspoon paprika

½ teaspoon dried oregano

⅛ teaspoon salt

Pinch cayenne pepper

Toss together the shrimp, chickpeas, bell pepper, onion, garlic, vinegar, olive oil, paprika, oregano, salt, and cayenne pepper in a large bowl. Taste, and adjust the seasonings.

INGREDIENT TIP: Additives that contain sodium are often added to shrimp in processing. Read the labels and look for a brand that contains lower amounts of sodium—less than 400 mg per 3-ounce serving.

PER SERVING: Calories: 338; Total Fat: 15g; Saturated Fat: 2g; Cholesterol: 83mg; Sodium: 510mg; Carbohydrates: 28g; Fiber: 7g; Added Sugars: 0g; Protein: 17g; Potassium: 455mg; Vitamin K: 12mcg

SPICY SHRIMP, FETA, AND WALNUT COUSCOUS

DASH • MEDITERRANEAN • ONE POT

Keep a bag of shrimp in the freezer, and you'll always have a quick, easy, lean, protein-rich food at the ready. Shrimp is higher in cholesterol than most fish, but a 3-ounce serving contains about the same amount of cholesterol as a single egg, so it's not a concern. Look for packaged shrimp with 400 mg or less cholesterol per 3-ounce serving. Thaw it overnight in the fridge in the package, or quick-thaw it loose in a bowl with a trickle of cold running water.

Serves 4

Hands-on time: 25 min

Total time: 30 min

1 tablespoon extra-virgin olive oil

2 cups frozen sliced onions and bell peppers

2 medium ripe tomatoes, chopped

2 garlic cloves, minced

1½ cups reduced-sodium chicken broth

½ teaspoon cayenne pepper

12 ounces sustainably sourced, frozen raw shrimp, thawed and peeled

1 cup uncooked whole-wheat couscous

⅓ cup chopped walnuts

⅓ cup crumbled feta cheese

1. Heat the oil in a large, heavy skillet over medium-high heat. When the oil is hot, add the onions and peppers. Cook, stirring occasionally, for 3 to 4 minutes.

2. Add the tomato and garlic, and cook for 1 minute. Add the chicken broth and cayenne pepper, and bring to a boil. Add the shrimp, and return to a boil.

3. Stir in the couscous. Remove the skillet from the heat, cover, and let stand until the couscous is tender and all the broth is absorbed, about 5 minutes.

4. Fluff with a fork. Top with the walnuts and feta cheese.

FLAVOR BOOST: If you like it spicier, add more cayenne. Top with chopped scallions.

PER SERVING: Calories: 392; Total Fat: 14g; Saturated Fat: 3g; Cholesterol: 150mg; Sodium: 490mg; Carbohydrates: 40g; Fiber: 5g; Added Sugars: g; Protein: 29g; Potassium: 680mg; Vitamin K: 10mcg

PAN-SEARED HALIBUT WITH CHIMICHURRI

Chimichurri is a flavorful Argentine, herb-based sauce traditionally served with grilled meat, but it also pairs well with a firm fish like halibut. Once you get comfortable with whipping up the Chimichurri, you can do it while the fish cooks. Pan-seared fish also goes well with Pineapple-Cranberry Salsa (page 183), Spicy Guacamole (page 156), or Tomato-Balsamic Vinaigrette (page 179).

Serves 4

Hands-on time: 10 min

Total time: 10 min

2 tablespoons extra-virgin olive oil

4 (5- to 6-ounce) sustainably sourced halibut fillets, fresh or thawed

1 recipe Chimichurri (page 180)

1. Heat the oil in a large, nonstick skillet over medium-high heat. When the oil is hot, sear the halibut for about 5 minutes on each side, until it flakes easily and is cooked to an internal temperature of 145°F.

2. Serve immediately, topped with the Chimichurri.

SUBSTITUTION TIP: Use this recipe with any thick, hearty fish fillet, such as cod, grouper, or red snapper.

PER SERVING: Calories: 371; Total Fat: 25g; Saturated Fat: 4g; Cholesterol: 112mg; Sodium: 248mg; Carbohydrates: 5g; Fiber: 1g; Added Sugars: 0g; Protein: 32g; Potassium: 763mg; Vitamin K: 78mcg

"HOME LATE" PANTRY TILAPIA WITH VEGGIE PASTA

DASH • MEDITERRANEAN • PORTABLE

This recipe will save you time when you get home late, because you can keep all the ingredients on hand. It works with flounder, sole, or any other thin white fish fillets. Leftovers make a great pasta salad for lunch. For a flavor boost, toss with an infused extra-virgin olive oil, such as garlic, lemon, or herbs. To mix it up, swap the olives for freshly grated Parmesan, Asiago, or goat cheese.

Serves 4

Hands-on time: 20 min

Total time: 20 min

8 ounces uncooked egg noodles

5 cups frozen vegetables of your choice

1 tablespoon canola or sunflower oil

1 pound sustainably sourced tilapia fillets, fresh or frozen and thawed

¼ teaspoon kosher salt

Freshly ground black pepper

1 tablespoon extra-virgin olive oil

1 teaspoon dried thyme, oregano, or basil *or* 1 tablespoon minced fresh herbs

10 kalamata olives, pitted and sliced (optional)

Zest and juice of 1 lemon (about 3 tablespoons lemon juice)

1. Preheat the oven to 450°F.

2. Fill a large a pot with water, and bring it to a boil over high heat. Cook the egg noodles to al dente, following the package directions. Add the frozen vegetables during the final 2 to 3 minutes of cooking.

3. While the pasta is cooking, lightly brush a rimmed baking sheet with canola oil. Lay the fish on it, and brush with the rest of the oil. Sprinkle with salt and pepper, and set aside.

4. When you're about to drain the pasta, put the fish in the oven. Bake until it just begins to flake at the edges, 4 to 5 minutes, depending on thickness. The center will still be a bit translucent, but the fish will continue to cook after you take it out of the oven.

5. Meanwhile, transfer the drained pasta and veggies to a large bowl, and toss with the olive oil, herbs, and olives (if using). Add the lemon zest and juice.

6. Use a fork to flake the cooked fish into the pasta.

INGREDIENT TIP: Canola and sunflower oils have high smoke points, meaning they can withstand high temperatures, up to about 460°F, before they start to burn and smoke. (Extra-virgin olive oil starts to smoke at about 410°F.) Other heart-healthy oils you can use at 450°F include grapeseed, light olive, and avocado.

PER SERVING: Calories: 462; Total Fat: 15g; Saturated Fat: 2g; Cholesterol: 100mg; Sodium: 419mg; Carbohydrates: 51g; Fiber: 7g; Added Sugars: 0g; Protein: 33g; Potassium: 750mg; Vitamin K: 68mcg

PECAN-CRUSTED CATFISH WITH ROASTED ROMAINE

DASH • MEDITERRANEAN

If you haven't tried roasted or grilled romaine hearts, you're in for a treat. Catfish has a dense flesh and a sweet, mild taste; you can substitute flounder, sole, tilapia, or any other sustainably sourced white fish. Thicker fillets may need more time; figure about 10 minutes per inch of thickness. Serve with wedges of lemon and cooked barley, brown rice, or crusty whole-wheat rolls, if you like.

Serves 4

Hands-on time: 20 min

Total time: 30 min

2 tablespoons extra-virgin olive oil, divided

2 hearts of romaine, halved lengthwise

1 garlic clove, minced

½ cup all-purpose flour

1 large egg

2 tablespoons water

¼ teaspoon paprika

½ cup very finely chopped pecans

12 ounces sustainably sourced catfish fillets, fresh or thawed

¼ teaspoon kosher salt

Freshly ground black pepper

1 lemon, cut into wedges

1. Preheat the oven to 425°F. Line two rimmed baking sheets with parchment paper, and drizzle each with ½ tablespoon of oil.

2. Lay the romaine halves, cut-side up, on one sheet, and drizzle with the remaining 1 tablespoon of oil. Sprinkle the romaine with the garlic.

3. Set the other sheet next to three wide bowls. Fill one bowl with the flour, beat the egg, water, and paprika together in the second bowl, and fill the last bowl with the pecans.

4. Pat the fish dry with a paper towel. Sprinkle with salt and pepper. Dip and flip each fillet in the flour, then the egg mixture, then the pecans. Lay on the baking sheet. Press any unused pecans into the fish.

5. Put both baking sheets in the oven and roast until the fish just starts to flake easily, 8 to 10 minutes. By then the romaine should be nicely browned. If not, remove the fish from the oven and broil the romaine for 2 to 3 minutes, watching carefully. Serve with lemon wedges.

SUBSTITUTION TIP: You can also use finely chopped walnuts or almonds as a coating for the fish.

PER SERVING: Calories: 367; Total Fat: 21g; Saturated Fat: 3g; Cholesterol: 96mg; Sodium: 80mg; Carbohydrates: 25g; Fiber: 8g; Added Sugars: 0g; Protein: 22g; Potassium: 1,186mg; Vitamin K: 326mcg

SOFRITO COD STEW

Sofrito is a sauce base used in Mediterranean and Latin American cooking. It varies by cuisine but typically includes finely chopped onion, bell pepper, and garlic cooked in olive oil with tomatoes. Substitute any white fish, such as tilapia or pollock, and any whole grain, such as farro.

Serves 4

Hands-on time: 30 min

Total time: 30 min

1 cup uncooked parboiled brown rice

¼ cup extra-virgin olive oil

1 large onion, finely chopped

1 green bell pepper, seeded and finely chopped

5 garlic cloves, minced

1 (28-ounce) can no-salt-added whole tomatoes

1 teaspoon dried thyme

¼ teaspoon salt

¼ teaspoon freshly ground black pepper

1 pound sustainably sourced cod fillets, fresh or thawed

½ teaspoon red pepper flakes (optional)

1. Cook the rice according to the package directions.

2. Meanwhile, heat the olive oil in a large skillet over medium heat. Add the onion, bell pepper, and garlic, and cook until softened, 5 to 7 minutes.

3. Turn up the heat, and add the tomatoes with their juice, thyme, salt, and black pepper. When it starts to boil, add the cod, pushing it down into the liquid, and turn down the heat so it simmers gently for 7 to 8 minutes.

4. Test the fish by flaking with a fork. If it flakes easily, separate it into bite-size pieces. If not, cook for a few more minutes.

5. Taste and adjust the seasonings, adding red pepper flakes if desired. Serve over the rice.

FLAVOR BOOST: Add ½ cup dry red or white wine along with the tomatoes in step 3.

LEFTOVERS: Whenever you cook a batch of whole grains, make extra; it freezes well. Defrost in the microwave at full power for 2 to 3 minutes, depending on the amount. Check and stir after 2 minutes.

PER SERVING: Calories: 449; Total Fat: 16g; Saturated Fat: 2g; Cholesterol: 492mg; Sodium: 233mg; Carbohydrates: 51g; Fiber: 6g; Added Sugars: 0g; Protein: 26g; Potassium: 1,077mg; Vitamin K: 21mcg

SEARED SCALLOPS AND LEMONY FENNEL

DASH • MEDITERRANEAN

Scallops are a treat, but they can be expensive. This dish also works well with other fish, and even with boneless, skinless chicken breasts cut into scallop-size pieces. The key with scallops is to not overcook them. They're done when both sides are seared and golden-brown and the sides look opaque.

Serves 4

Hands-on time: 20 min

Total time: 30 min

1 cup uncooked
pearl barley

2 cups reduced-sodium
chicken broth

2 tablespoons extra-virgin
olive oil, divided

2 large fennel bulbs, very
thinly sliced

½ red bell pepper, chopped

2 shallots, minced

2 garlic cloves, minced

1 pound sustainably
sourced sea scallops, fresh
or thawed

Freshly ground black
pepper (optional)

1 tablespoon minced fresh
or dried flat-leaf parsley
(optional)

Zest and juice of 1 lemon
(about 3 tablespoons juice)

1. Cook the barley until tender, according to the package directions, using the chicken broth instead of water.

2. Heat a large skillet over medium-high heat. Add 1 tablespoon of oil. When the oil is hot, add the fennel, pepper, shallots, and garlic. Sauté until the fennel is tender and lightly browned, 5 to 6 minutes. Transfer to a bowl to keep warm.

3. When the barley is 5 minutes from being ready, add the remaining 1 tablespoon of oil to the skillet. Add the scallops, and sprinkle with pepper, if desired. Cook until the scallops are browned on both sides, about 2 minutes per side.

4. Spoon a bed of barley onto each plate, top with the fennel mixture, then add the scallops. Top with parsley, lemon zest and juice, and more black pepper, if desired.

FLAVOR BOOST: Top with a handful of toasted slivered almonds, for added flavor and a bit of crunch.

PER SERVING: Calories: 377; Total Fat: 9g; Saturated Fat: 1g; Cholesterol: 29mg; Sodium: 566mg; Carbohydrates: 55g; Fiber: 12g; Added Sugars: 0g; Protein: 22g; Potassium: 1,024mg; Vitamin K: 95mcg

ROSEMARY-LEMON SALMON

MEDITERRANEAN • ONE POT

You can pair this simple salmon with just about any salad or side dish in chapter 3. Or substitute steelhead trout if you like. If you use farmed salmon or steelhead trout, which are typically high in fat (mostly heart-healthy omega-3s), you can skip the olive oil in the recipe. Wild salmon is typically leaner and benefits from the extra moisture.

Serves 4

Hands-on time: 10 min

Total time: 25 min

1 pound sustainably sourced fresh, skin-on salmon fillets

Zest and juice of
½ lemon (about
1½ tablespoons juice)

1 garlic clove, minced

¼ teaspoon kosher salt

Freshly ground
black pepper

2 fresh rosemary sprigs *or*
1 teaspoon dried rosemary

1 tablespoon extra-virgin olive oil (optional)

1. Set the oven rack to the second-highest level, and preheat the broiler.

2. Line a rimmed baking sheet with aluminum foil. Place the salmon, skin-side down, on the sheet. Top with the lemon zest and juice, garlic, salt, and pepper. Lay the rosemary sprigs on top. Drizzle with olive oil (if using).

3. Broil the salmon for 5 minutes, then move to a lower rack and reduce the heat to 325°F.

4. Cook for another 8 to 10 minutes, until the salmon is nearly done (see the Cooking Tip). Let the fish rest, tented with foil, for 5 minutes before serving.

COOKING TIP: Salmon is delicious when it's not over-cooked. A meat thermometer inserted into the thickest part should measure just 125°F when you take it out. Tent with foil and let it rest until the fish reaches 145°F. It should look slightly translucent when you pull it from the oven, and opaque after resting.

PER SERVING: Calories: 193; Total Fat: 11g; Saturated Fat: 2g; Cholesterol: 62mg; Sodium: 171mg; Carbohydrates: 1g; Fiber: 0g; Added Sugars: 0g; Protein: 23g; Potassium: 564mg; Vitamin K: 2mcg

CHILI SALMON SHEET PAN DINNER

DASH • MEDITERRANEAN

This is one of my favorite ways to cook salmon. The whole meal cooks in the oven, leaving time to set the table, tidy the kitchen, and breathe. The spice rub works well for chicken or pork tenderloin, too. I often bring a batch of this spice mix in a zip-top bag on vacation if we're staying somewhere with a kitchen. Then, I just pick up fresh fish and vegetables for a no-fuss dinner.

Serves 4

Hands-on time: 20 min

Total time: 30 min

1½ tablespoons chili powder

½ teaspoon dried oregano

¼ teaspoon kosher salt

1 large sweet potato, scrubbed and cut into ¾-inch cubes

2 tablespoons canola or sunflower oil, divided

1 head broccoli, cut into florets, or 2 cups frozen broccoli florets

1 pound sustainably sourced salmon fillets, fresh or thawed

1. Preheat the oven to 420°F. Line two rimmed baking sheets with parchment paper.

2. Mix the chili powder, oregano, and salt in a small bowl.

3. Toss the sweet potato in a large bowl with 1 tablespoon of oil and 1 teaspoon of seasoning mix. Spread out on one baking sheet, and slide into the oven.

4. In the same bowl, toss the broccoli with the remaining 1 tablespoon of oil and another 1 teaspoon of seasoning. Spread out on the other baking sheet, and put in the oven. Set a timer for 5 minutes.

5. Rub the remainder of the seasoning mix onto the salmon. When the timer goes off, toss the sweet potatoes and broccoli. Slide them over, and add the salmon to the sheet pans.

6. Remove the salmon from the sheet pans when it is nearly done (see Cooking Tip, page 112), 8 to 10 minutes, depending on thickness, and tent with foil. Keep roasting the vegetables until they are as crisp as you like them, about 5 minutes more.

PER SERVING: Calories: 317; Total Fat: 14g; Saturated Fat: 2g; Cholesterol: 62mg; Sodium: 233mg; Carbohydrates: 21g; Fiber: 4g; Added Sugars: 0g; Protein: 25g; Potassium: 1,001mg; Vitamin K: 8mcg

TOMATO AND ZUCCHINI WITH SALMON AND FARRO

DASH • MEDITERRANEAN

Farro is growing in popularity, thanks to its nutty flavor and nutrients, which include high amounts of fiber and protein. It typically takes less than half an hour to cook, which is faster than brown rice. If you spiralize the zucchini, make a lengthwise slit in it first so the noodles are short and manageable. And for a boost of added flavor, sprinkle the finished dish with freshly ground black pepper and red pepper flakes.

Serves 4

Hands-on time: 25 min

Total time: 25 min

1 cup uncooked farro

2 tablespoons extra-virgin olive oil

4 shallots, thinly sliced

2 cups cherry tomatoes, halved

1 teaspoon dried thyme

1 medium zucchini

2 garlic cloves

Zest and juice of 1 lemon (about 3 tablespoons juice)

1 (7.5-ounce) can wild salmon, drained

4 cups baby spinach

½ cup crumbled feta cheese

1. Cook the farro according to the package directions.

2. Meanwhile, heat the oil in a large skillet over medium heat. Add the shallots, tomatoes, and thyme. Cook until the shallots start to brown, 5 or 6 minutes.

3. While that's cooking, grate or spiralize the zucchini and mince the garlic.

4. Add the zucchini, garlic, and lemon zest and juice to the skillet with the tomatoes, and cook for a few minutes, stirring occasionally.

5. Drain the salmon, reserving 1 tablespoon of the liquid from the can. Add the salmon to the skillet, along with the reserved canning liquid. Break the fish apart with a fork. Add the cooked farro and the spinach. Stir everything together to heat through.

6. Taste and adjust the seasonings. Top with the feta cheese.

LEFTOVERS: If you use only part of a can of salmon, you can freeze the remaining salmon for up to 3 months. Defrost overnight in the refrigerator.

PER SERVING: Calories: 405; Total Fat: 15g; Saturated Fat: 4g; Cholesterol: 52mg; Sodium: 411mg; Carbohydrates: 43g; Fiber: 7g; Added Sugars: 0g; Protein: 26g; Potassium: 955mg; Vitamin K: 139mcg

GRILLED SALMON TACO PARTY

DASH · MEDITERRANEAN

Who doesn't love a good fish taco? You can make this recipe's yogurt-salsa sauce with jarred salsa, but fresh will taste better. You can also swap in sour cream for the yogurt.

Serves 4

Hands-on time: 25 min

Total time: 30 min

For the salmon

2 tablespoons canola or sunflower oil

2 tablespoons reduced-sodium tamari

2 tablespoons freshly squeezed lime juice

1 tablespoon ground cumin

2 garlic cloves, minced

1 pound sustainably sourced, thin, skin-on salmon fillets, fresh or thawed

For the tacos

⅔ cup plain yogurt

2 tablespoons Fresh Tomato Salsa (page 182) or lower-sodium store-bought salsa

½ cup chopped fresh cilantro

1½ cups coleslaw veggie mix

1 avocado, peeled, pitted, and sliced

12 corn tortillas

1. Preheat the grill to medium-high. (Alternatively, preheat the oven to 400°F and line a rimmed baking sheet with aluminum foil.)

2. To marinate the salmon, mix the oil, tamari, lime juice, cumin, and garlic in a flat dish, and add the salmon. Let it marinate for at least 10 minutes, turning halfway.

3. Remove the salmon from the marinade and place it, skin-side down, on the grill. Cover the grill and cook, undisturbed, until the flesh flakes easily, 8 to 10 minutes. Use a spatula to remove the fish from the grill and gently flake it into smaller pieces. (If you're cooking it in the oven, remove the salmon from the marinade and place the fish on the baking sheet. Bake for 10 to 15 minutes, depending on the thickness.)

4. Meanwhile, mix the yogurt and salsa together in a bowl. Put out the cilantro, coleslaw mix, and sliced avocado in their own bowls.

5. Wrap the tortillas in a clean, damp dish towel or paper towel and microwave for 30 to 60 seconds. Serve with the salmon and taco fillings.

COOKING TIP: If you don't have a microwave, heat the tortillas, two at a time, in a lightly oiled skillet.

PER SERVING: Calories: 490; Total Fat: 22g; Saturated Fat: 3g; Cholesterol: 65mg; Sodium: 503mg; Carbohydrates: 42g; Fiber: 8g; Added Sugars: 0g; Protein: 31g; Potassium: 1,061mg; Vitamin K: 40mcg

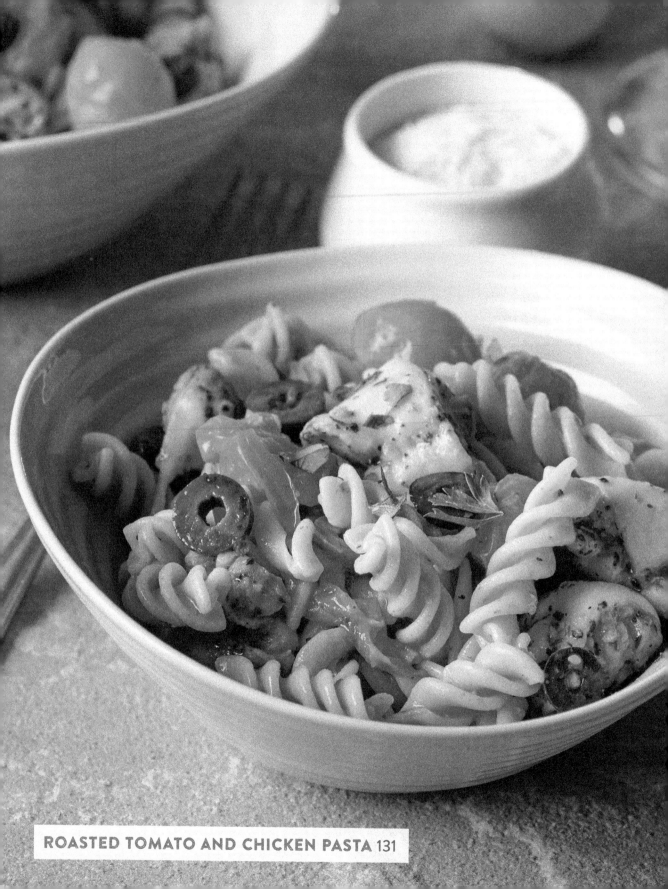

ROASTED TOMATO AND CHICKEN PASTA 131

CHAPTER SIX

POULTRY ENTRÉES

PAN-SEARED CHICKEN

MEDITERRANEAN • 5-INGREDIENT • ONE POT • PORTABLE

This simple chicken dish pairs well with any of the green salads in chapter 3. You can prepare the salad while the chicken cooks. If you prefer dark meat, you can make this recipe with boneless, skinless chicken thighs. They're juicier but not much higher in saturated fat, especially if you trim them before cooking.

Serves 4

Hands-on time: 10 min

Total time: 20 min

1 pound boneless, skinless chicken breasts

¼ teaspoon kosher salt

Freshly ground black pepper

2 tablespoons canola or sunflower oil

1. Pat the chicken dry with paper towels. Season with the salt and pepper.

2. Heat a large, heavy skillet over medium-high heat. Add the canola or sunflower oil. When the oil is hot (a drop of water should sizzle), add the chicken—make sure there is oil under each piece. Cover the pan.

3. After 5 minutes, check that the undersides are crispy and golden, and flip them over. If they feel stuck, give them another minute or two.

4. Cover and cook the other side for 5 minutes more, without disturbing the chicken. Use a meat thermometer to ensure that it has reached 165°F inside. It should be opaque with mostly clear juices. Transfer the chicken to a cutting board. Let it rest for a few minutes before slicing.

PER SERVING: Calories: 198; Total Fat: 10g; Saturated Fat: 1g; Cholesterol: 83mg; Sodium: 171mg; Carbohydrates: 0g; Fiber: 0g; Added Sugars: 0g; Protein: 26g; Potassium: 379mg; Vitamin K: 5mcg

GRILLED GARLIC-LIME CHICKEN

MEDITERRANEAN • 5-INGREDIENT • ONE POT • PORTABLE

This dish pairs perfectly with Pineapple-Cranberry Salsa (page 183) or with one of the salads or vegetarian entrées in chapters 3 and 4. The longer you can marinate the chicken, the better, but even 10 minutes will give the flavors a chance to develop. Add a chopped jalapeño pepper to the marinade for an extra kick.

Serves 4

Hands-on time: 20 min

Total time: 30 min

1 pound boneless, skinless chicken breasts

2 tablespoons canola or sunflower oil, plus more for oiling the grill

Zest and juice of 1 lime

2 garlic cloves, minced

Freshly ground black pepper

To cook on a grill

1. Preheat the grill to medium-high.

2. Arrange the chicken in a single layer in a shallow dish. Drizzle with the oil and lime juice. Sprinkle with the lime zest. Top with the garlic and pepper. Toss gently to mix the flavors and coat the chicken. Let the chicken marinate for at least 10 minutes.

3. Lightly coat the grill rack with oil. Transfer the chicken to the grill and cook until a meat thermometer reads 165°F, 4 to 5 minutes on each side. It should be opaque with mostly clear juices. Allow the chicken to rest for at least 5 minutes before cutting it.

→

To cook under the broiler

1. Set an oven rack 4 to 5 inches from the broiler, and preheat the broiler to high. Line a rimmed baking sheet with aluminum foil.

2. Cut each breast in half horizontally to make 2 thin cutlets. Press down to flatten. Arrange the chicken in a single layer in a shallow dish. Drizzle with the oil and lime juice. Sprinkle with the lime zest. Top with the garlic and pepper. Toss gently to mix the flavors and coat the chicken. Let the chicken marinate for at least 10 minutes.

3. Transfer the cutlets to the baking sheet. Broil, turning once, until the chicken is lightly browned on both sides and cooked to an internal temperature of 165°F, 4 to 5 minutes per side. It should be opaque with mostly clear juices. Allow the chicken to rest for at least 5 minutes before cutting it.

PER SERVING: Calories: 202; Total Fat: 10g; Saturated Fat: 1g; Cholesterol: 83mg; Sodium: 51mg; Carbohydrates: 1g; Fiber: 0g; Added Sugars: 0g; Protein: 26g; Potassium: 394mg; Vitamin K: 5mcg

ARUGULA PASTA SALAD WITH CHICKEN

DASH • MEDITERRANEAN • PORTABLE

This recipe is a simple way to use leftover cooked chicken, such as Pan-Seared Chicken (page 120). Or substitute salmon or white beans for a different main dish. You could also leave out the protein entirely to make a satisfying side dish. The strong flavors in this salad can stand up to whole-wheat penne, but if you prefer, use regular pasta.

Serves 4

Hands-on time: 15 min

Total time: 15 min

8 ounces uncooked whole-wheat penne

2 cups chopped cooked chicken

1 (5-ounce) package arugula, trimmed of large stems and torn into bite-size pieces if necessary

½ cup sliced Simple Roasted Peppers (page 61) or jarred roasted red peppers

2 tablespoons extra-virgin olive oil

Zest and juice of 1 lemon (about 3 tablespoons juice)

⅓ cup grated Parmesan cheese

Freshly ground black pepper (optional)

1. Cook the pasta to al dente according to the package directions. When it's finished, drain and rinse with cool water.

2. Meanwhile, mix the chicken, arugula, roasted peppers, oil, and lemon zest and juice in a large salad bowl.

3. Add the pasta and toss gently to combine. Top with the cheese and black pepper, if you like.

FLAVOR BOOST: For a flavorful veggie boost, add 2 heads of Belgian endive, trimmed and thinly sliced.

PER SERVING: Calories: 433; Total Fat: 18g; Saturated Fat: 3g; Cholesterol: 15mg; Sodium: 236mg; Carbohydrates: 46g; Fiber: 7g; Added Sugars: 0g; Protein: 26g; Potassium: 676mg; Vitamin K: 49mcg

PESTO, ASPARAGUS, AND CHICKEN PASTA

DASH • MEDITERRANEAN • PORTABLE

Pesto is wonderful with chicken (or fish) and pasta, and this dish takes care of the vegetables for the night, too. Mix it up with the veggies, if you like: Use broccoli instead of asparagus. Even frozen works! Enjoy the leftovers as a cold pasta salad the next day, or reheat them in the microwave.

Serves 4

Hands-on time: 15 min

Total time: 15 min

8 ounces uncooked bowtie pasta

1 pound asparagus

1 tablespoon extra-virgin olive oil

12 ounces boneless, skinless chicken breasts, cut into bite-size pieces

½ cup Walnut Pesto (page 181)

2 medium ripe tomatoes, chopped

¼ cup grated Parmesan cheese (optional)

1. Start cooking the pasta, setting a timer for 4 minutes less than the al dente cooking time printed on the package. Remove the woody ends of the asparagus, and cut the spears into 1-inch pieces. When the timer goes off, scoop out ½ cup of cooking water and add the asparagus to the pasta pot. Bring the water back to a boil, and set the timer for 4 more minutes.

2. Meanwhile, heat the oil in a large skillet over medium-high heat. Sauté the chicken until it's cooked through, 5 to 10 minutes. It should be opaque with mostly clear juices. Stir in the tomatoes, and remove the skillet from the heat.

3. Drain the pasta and asparagus, and return them to the pasta pot. Toss with the pesto and ¼ cup of the reserved cooking water. Add the chicken, tomatoes, and more cooking water if it seems dry. Top with the Parmesan, if desired.

INGREDIENT TIP: Use store-bought pesto if you like, but use just ⅓ cup and perk it up with minced fresh basil, if possible.

PER SERVING: Calories: 485; Total Fat: 17g; Saturated Fat: 4g; Cholesterol: 68mg; Sodium: 201mg; Carbohydrates: 50g; Fiber: 5g; Added Sugars: 0g; Protein: 33g; Potassium: 821mg; Vitamin K: 84mcg

CHILI CHICKEN, PEPPERS, AND CORN

DASH • MEDITERRANEAN

If you're in the mood for hearty comfort food, look no further. The peanut sauce contributes protein in addition to healthy fats, so you can go light on the chicken and heavy on the veggies.

Serves 4

Hands-on time: 30 min

Total time: 30 min

¾ cup uncooked parboiled brown rice

2 tablespoons canola or sunflower oil, divided

5 cups frozen sliced bell peppers and onions

¼ teaspoon kosher salt (optional)

Freshly ground black pepper (optional)

12 ounces boneless, skinless chicken breasts, cut into bite-size pieces

1½ cups reduced-sodium chicken broth

⅓ cup natural peanut butter (smooth or crunchy)

2 tablespoons chili powder

1 teaspoon dried tarragon

1 cup frozen corn kernels

Juice of 1 lime (about 2 tablespoons)

½ cup chopped fresh cilantro

1. Cook the rice according to the package directions.

2. Meanwhile, heat 1 tablespoon of oil in a large skillet over medium-high heat. When it is hot, add the peppers and onions. Sprinkle with salt and pepper (if using). Cook, stirring frequently, until they soften, 3 to 4 minutes. Transfer to a plate.

3. Add the remaining 1 tablespoon of oil and the chicken to the skillet. Sauté until the chicken is cooked through, 5 to 10 minutes. It should be opaque with mostly clear juices. Transfer to the plate with the vegetables.

4. Add the chicken broth, peanut butter, chili powder, and tarragon to the pan, stirring to mix. When the sauce comes together, add the corn. When it is hot, mix the chicken and vegetables back in.

5. Remove from the heat, and stir in the lime juice and cilantro. Serve over the rice.

FLAVOR BOOST: Scatter some fresh salsa, chopped jalapeño pepper, or diced avocado on top.

PER SERVING: Calories: 521; Total Fat: 22g; Saturated Fat: 3g; Cholesterol: 64mg; Sodium: 213mg; Carbohydrates: 54g; Fiber: 7g; Added Sugars: 0g; Protein: 31g; Potassium: 977mg; Vitamin K: 16mcg

ALMOST CHICKEN PARMESAN

DASH • MEDITERRANEAN

Here's a simpler but still satisfying take on the original. Traditionally, this is served over spaghetti, but it's also a good topping for spaghetti squash (cooked as for Spaghetti Squash with Walnuts and Parmesan, page 70) or lightly sautéed zucchini noodles.

Serves 4

Hands-on time: 20 min

Total time: 30 min

3 to 4 medium tomatoes, cut into wedges

3 tablespoons extra-virgin olive oil, divided

¼ teaspoon kosher salt (optional)

1 pound chicken breast cutlets or tenders

½ cup whole-wheat panko breadcrumbs

½ cup grated Parmesan cheese, divided

2 tablespoons ground flaxseed

½ teaspoon paprika

½ teaspoon garlic powder

½ teaspoon ground mustard

¼ teaspoon freshly ground black pepper

1. Preheat the oven to 400°F.

2. Scatter the tomatoes on a rimmed baking sheet, and drizzle with 1 tablespoon of oil. Sprinkle with salt (if using), and slide them into the oven so they can get a head start on roasting.

3. Meanwhile, line a second baking sheet with parchment paper. Line up the chicken pieces on it, and rub with 1 tablespoon of oil.

4. In a medium bowl, mix the panko, ¼ cup of Parmesan, flaxseed, paprika, garlic powder, ground mustard, and black pepper. Spread over the chicken. Drizzle the remaining 1 tablespoon of oil over the top.

5. Bake until the chicken is cooked through, about 20 minutes. Start checking after 15 minutes so you don't overcook it. It should be opaque with mostly clear juices. When the chicken is done, the tomatoes should be starting to brown.

6. Serve the chicken topped with the tomatoes and the remaining ¼ cup of Parmesan cheese.

COOKING TIP: Chicken breast cutlets and tenders are thin, quick-cooking pieces. If you have full chicken breasts, slice them horizontally and press down to flatten.

PER SERVING: Calories: 343; Total Fat: 18g; Saturated Fat: 4g; Cholesterol: 91mg; Sodium: 370mg; Carbohydrates: 14g; Fiber: 3g; Added Sugars: 0g; Protein: 32g; Potassium: 693mg; Vitamin K: 15mcg

ARTICHOKE AND ZUCCHINI CHICKEN THIGHS

DASH • MEDITERRANEAN

Delicious marinated artichoke hearts can be high in sodium, but much of it is drained away with the liquid in the jar or can. The other ingredients in this recipe are low in sodium to balance it. For an extra flavor boost, add a splash of dry white wine when you add the artichokes.

Serves 4

Hands-on time: 20 min

Total time: 20 min

1 cup uncooked quinoa

2 teaspoons unsalted butter

1 pound boneless, skinless chicken thighs, cut into bite-size pieces

2 medium zucchini, cut into bite-size pieces

1 garlic clove, minced (optional)

1 (12-ounce) jar quartered marinated artichoke hearts, drained

1 tablespoon freshly squeezed lemon juice

¼ cup grated Parmesan cheese (optional)

¼ cup minced fresh flat-leaf parsley (optional)

1. Cook the quinoa according to the package directions.

2. Meanwhile, heat the butter in a large skillet over medium-high heat. When the butter is hot, add the chicken and cook until brown, about 2 minutes on each side. Add the zucchini and garlic (if using), and cook until the chicken and zucchini are cooked through, 5 to 10 minutes. The chicken should be opaque with mostly clear juices. Add the artichoke hearts and cook just long enough to warm them up.

3. Remove from the heat and sprinkle with the lemon juice, cheese, and parsley (if using). Serve over the quinoa.

PER SERVING: Calories: 388; Total Fat: 11g; Saturated Fat: 4g; Cholesterol: 115mg; Sodium: 429mg; Carbohydrates: 39g; Fiber: 8g; Added Sugars: 0g; Protein: 34g; Potassium: 1,025mg; Vitamin K: 80mcg

WEEKNIGHT COQ AU VIN

DASH • MEDITERRANEAN • ONE POT

This isn't quite the long-simmering classic, but it's a pretty good approximation for those nights when time is short. Add garlic or a sprig of rosemary along with the thyme in step 2 for more flavor. Serve with roasted vegetables, mashed potatoes, pasta, wild rice, or a light salad.

Serves 4

Hands-on time: 25 min

Total time: 30 min

2 tablespoons Better Butter (page 176) *or* 1 tablespoon unsalted butter plus
1 tablespoon extra-virgin olive oil

1 pound boneless, skinless chicken thighs, pounded to ½-inch thickness

¼ teaspoon kosher salt

Freshly ground
black pepper

3 large carrots, peeled and thinly sliced on the diagonal

8 ounces sliced mushrooms

1 yellow onion, sliced

1 cup dry red wine

1 cup reduced-sodium chicken broth

1 tablespoon tomato paste

3 fresh thyme sprigs

1. Melt the Better Butter in a heavy skillet over medium-high heat. Sprinkle the chicken with salt and pepper. When the butter starts to froth, add the chicken, and brown for 1 to 2 minutes on each side. Transfer to a plate.

2. Add the carrots, mushrooms, and onion to the skillet. Sauté until the onion starts to soften, 3 to 4 minutes, then add the wine, broth, tomato paste, and thyme. Cook until the vegetables are just crisp-tender, 7 to 8 minutes.

3. Return the chicken to the pan, and simmer until cooked through, 5 to 10 minutes. It should be opaque with mostly clear juices. Remove the thyme and serve.

COOKING TIP: Pounding chicken helps it cook evenly. Place one piece at a time in a large, zip-top bag on a cutting board, and whack them all over until they are an even thickness. A heavy skillet, rolling pin, or meat mallet will do the job. If you use chicken breasts, slice them horizontally into thin cutlets so they cook more quickly.

PER SERVING: Calories: 296; Total Fat: 12g; Saturated Fat: 3g; Cholesterol: 115mg; Sodium: 295mg; Carbohydrates: 11g; Fiber: 2g; Added Sugars: 0g; Protein: 26g; Potassium: 801mg; Vitamin K: 13mcg

SUN-DRIED TOMATO TURKEY BURGERS

ONE POT

People who say turkey burgers are too dry clearly haven't tried this recipe, which swaps the saturated fat in a typical burger for the heart-healthier fats of oil-packed sun-dried tomatoes and avocado. These burgers are also great on the grill. Serve them on whole-wheat buns with a simple salad or crunchy raw vegetables and hummus. For bigger appetites, pair the burgers with Roasted Sweet Potatoes (page 68).

Serves 6

Hands-on time: 30 min

Total time: 30 min

1 pound ground turkey

½ cup rolled oats

¼ cup sun-dried tomatoes in oil, drained and chopped

¼ cup finely chopped red onion

¼ cup chopped fresh cilantro

2 garlic cloves, minced

6 whole-wheat hamburger buns

1 avocado, peeled, pitted, and sliced

6 lettuce leaves (optional)

6 tomato slices (optional)

1. Set an oven rack about 3 inches from the broiler, and preheat the broiler. Line a rimmed baking sheet with aluminum foil.

2. In a large bowl, mix the turkey with the oats, sun-dried tomatoes, onion, cilantro, and garlic. Shape into 6 (½-inch-thick) patties.

3. Place the patties on the baking sheet, and broil for 3 to 4 minutes on each side. If you want to be sure they're done, slide an instant-read thermometer into the side of a burger. It should read 165°F.

4. While the burgers are cooking, prepare a serving platter with the buns, avocado, lettuce, and tomato (if using). Let people assemble their own burgers.

SUBSTITUTION TIP: Top with Swiss or goat cheese if you don't have a ripe avocado.

PER SERVING: Calories: 366; Total Fat: 15g; Saturated Fat: 3g; Cholesterol: 52mg; Sodium: 353mg; Carbohydrates: 35g; Fiber: 6g; Added Sugars: 0g; Protein: 24g; Potassium: 620mg; Vitamin K: 21mcg

GRILLED SUMMER SQUASH AND CHICKEN WITH FARRO

DASH • MEDITERRANEAN • PORTABLE

This recipe is a delicious way to use leftover cooked chicken. If you don't have any on hand, pick up a rotisserie chicken or grill a couple of chicken breasts along with the vegetables (see Grilled Garlic-Lime Chicken, page 121). Use fresh dill or tarragon in place of the parsley for a different flavor.

Serves 4

Hands-on time: 30 min

Total time: 30 min

3 tablespoons extra-virgin olive oil, plus more for oiling the baking sheet

1¼ cups uncooked farro

1 large sweet onion, cut into 3 or 4 thick slices

2 pounds (about 8 small) assorted summer squash, cut lengthwise into ½-inch-thick slices

1½ cups bite-size cooked chicken pieces

¼ cup crumbled goat cheese

¼ cup chopped walnuts

¼ cup chopped fresh flat-leaf parsley (optional)

2 tablespoons freshly squeezed lemon juice

½ teaspoon kosher salt, divided

Freshly ground black pepper

1. Preheat the grill to medium high. (Alternatively, preheat the oven to 425°F and brush a rimmed baking sheet with a thin layer of oil.)

2. Cook the farro according to the package directions.

3. Meanwhile, brush the onion and squash slices on both sides with the oil. Place the onion and squash slices on the grill (or baking sheet in the oven). Grill until the vegetables are golden brown, about 15 minutes, flipping the slices halfway through.

4. Meanwhile, in a large bowl, combine the chicken, goat cheese, walnuts, parsley (if using), lemon juice, and any remaining olive oil. Season with salt and pepper. Add the cooked farro.

5. When the onion and squash slices are golden brown, transfer them to a cutting board. Cut into 1-inch pieces, and toss with the salad.

SUBSTITUTION TIP: Substitute pasta, quinoa, or rice for the farro if you have some on hand. This is a good way to use up leftover cooked whole grains.

PER SERVING: Calories: 510; Total Fat: 24g; Saturated Fat: 4g; Cholesterol: 42mg; Sodium: 327mg; Carbohydrates: 52g; Fiber: 8g; Added Sugars: 0g; Protein: 25g; Potassium: 1,119mg; Vitamin K: 80mcg

ROASTED TOMATO AND CHICKEN PASTA

DASH • MEDITERRANEAN

This simple weeknight dish is made with chicken thighs because they're more forgiving than breasts. They're a bit higher in saturated fat, but not much. The bold flavors can stand up to whole-wheat pasta, but use regular if you prefer. Roast a sheet of asparagus, bell peppers, or other veggies tossed in oil while you're at it, and just stir them in. Finish with fresh parsley, basil, thyme, or oregano if you have some on hand.

Serves 4

Hands-on time: 20 min

Total time: 30 min

1 pound boneless, skinless chicken thighs, cut into bite-size pieces

1/8 teaspoon kosher salt (optional)

1/4 teaspoon freshly ground black pepper (optional)

4 cups cherry tomatoes, halved

4 garlic cloves, minced

1 tablespoon canola or sunflower oil

1 teaspoon dried basil

8 ounces uncooked whole-wheat rotini

10 kalamata olives, pitted and sliced

1/4 teaspoon red pepper flakes (optional)

1/4 cup grated Parmesan cheese (optional)

1. Preheat the oven to 450°F.

2. Season the chicken with salt and pepper, if desired. Toss the chicken in a large bowl with the tomatoes, garlic, oil, and basil. Transfer to a rimmed baking sheet, and spread out evenly.

3. Roast until the chicken is cooked through, 15 to 20 minutes, tossing halfway though. A meat thermometer should read 165°F.

4. Meanwhile, cook the pasta to al dente according to the package directions. Drain.

5. In a large serving bowl, toss the chicken and tomatoes with the pasta, olives, and pepper flakes (if using). Top with Parmesan, if desired.

COOKING TIP: Olives off the tree contain a bitter compound that is fermented out using a salt-based brine—which is why olives are always a bit salty. If you don't add the olives here, double the salt.

PER SERVING: Calories: 458; Total Fat: 14g; Saturated Fat: 3g; Cholesterol: 110mg; Sodium: 441mg; Carbohydrates: 52g; Fiber: 8g; Added Sugars: 0g; Protein: 34g; Potassium: 968mg; Vitamin K: 24mcg

OAT RISOTTO WITH MUSHROOMS, KALE, AND CHICKEN

DASH • MEDITERRANEAN

Oats aren't just for breakfast! Savory dishes made with oats are growing in popularity, and for good reason: Oats are a whole-grain, delicious, affordable comfort food. There is a dizzying array of oat products. Steel-cut oats are whole oat kernels cut into pieces. Old-fashioned or rolled oats are flattened oat kernels. Quick or minute oats are flattened and pre-cooked. Instant oats are rolled very thin, precooked, and usually come in packets with sugar, sodium, and flavorings.

Serves 4

Hands-on time: 30 min

Total time: 30 min

4 cups reduced-sodium chicken broth

1 tablespoon extra-virgin olive oil

1 small onion, finely chopped

1 pound sliced mushrooms

1 pound boneless, skinless chicken thighs, cut into bite-size pieces

1¼ cups quick-cooking steel-cut oats

1 (10-ounce) package frozen chopped kale (about 4 cups)

½ cup grated Parmesan cheese (optional)

Freshly ground black pepper (optional)

1. In a medium saucepan, bring the broth to a simmer over medium-low heat.

2. Warm the olive oil in a large, nonstick skillet over medium-high heat. Sauté the onion and mushrooms until the onion is translucent, about 5 minutes. Push the vegetables to the side, and add the chicken. Let it sit untouched until it browns, about 2 minutes.

3. Add the oats. Cook for 1 minute, stirring constantly. Add ½ cup of the hot broth, and stir until it is completely absorbed. Continue stirring in broth, ½ cup at a time, until it is absorbed and the oats and chicken are cooked, about 10 minutes. If you run out of broth, switch to hot water.

4. Stir in the frozen kale, and cook until it's warm. Top with Parmesan and black pepper, if you like.

Garnish with minced parsley and red pepper flakes. You can also substitute ½ cup dry white wine for ½ cup of the chicken broth.

All varieties of oats have similar amounts of fiber, vitamins, and minerals. The main difference is in how quickly they're digested, with the steel-cut and old-fashioned/rolled oats breaking down more slowly, which is helpful for blood sugar control. The quick-cooking steel-cut oats used in this risotto are simply cut into smaller pieces, enabling you to make this dish in under 30 minutes.

PER SERVING: Calories: 470; Total Fat: 16g; Saturated Fat: 4g; Cholesterol: 118mg; Sodium: 389mg; Carbohydrates: 44g; Fiber: 9g; Added Sugars: g; Protein: 40g; Potassium: 1,351mg; Vitamin K: 534mcg

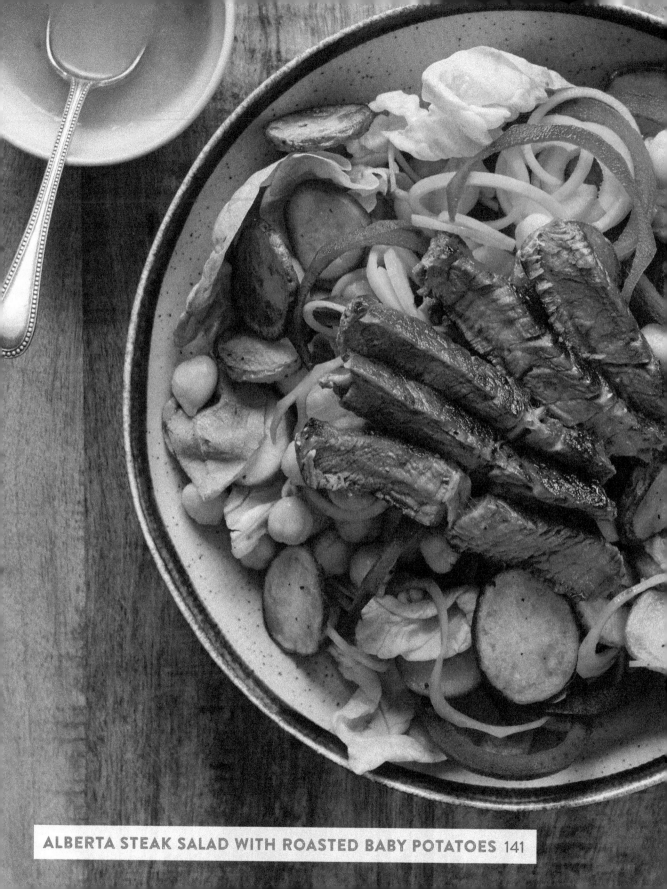

ALBERTA STEAK SALAD WITH ROASTED BABY POTATOES 141

MEAT ENTRÉES

BEEF AND CORN FIESTA SALAD

DASH • ONE POT • PORTABLE

Start with this basic recipe, and add anything else you love and/or want to use up: finely chopped red onion, fresh cilantro, and slivers of carrot or bell pepper all work well. Jazz it up with Spicy Guacamole (page 156), Fresh Tomato Salsa (page 182), sour cream, Baked Tortilla Chips (page 155), or a squeeze of fresh lime juice.

Serves 4

Hands-on time: 25 min

Total time: 25 min

2 cups frozen corn kernels

8 ounces extra-lean (7% fat) ground beef

¼ teaspoon kosher salt

Freshly ground black pepper (optional)

1 small onion, chopped

1 (15-ounce) can no-salt-added kidney beans, rinsed and drained

1 (14-ounce) can no-salt-added diced tomatoes

1 teaspoon chili powder

1 teaspoon ground cumin

4 cups torn romaine lettuce

2 medium tomatoes, chopped

1 avocado, peeled, pitted, and sliced

½ cup shredded Cheddar cheese

1. Put the corn in a large salad bowl to let it thaw.

2. Meanwhile, place a large sauté pan over medium heat. When it's hot, add the beef. Season with salt and pepper, if desired. Do not touch for 2–3 minutes, until the bottom is nicely browned.

3. Add the onion, and continue to brown the meat, stirring to cook on all sides. When it is no longer pink, add the beans, canned tomatoes with their juice, chili powder, and cumin. Simmer for 5 minutes.

4. Add the lettuce and fresh tomatoes to the salad bowl, and toss. Add the avocado slices on one side of the salad. Add the beef mixture on the other side. Sprinkle with the cheese.

SUBSTITUTION TIP: To make this salad vegetarian, substitute shelled toasted pumpkin seeds for the beef. Just sauté the onion and gently warm the beans and canned tomatoes with the chili and cumin, then stir in the pumpkin seeds. For a vegan salad, leave off the cheese, too, and add a sprinkle of nutritional yeast instead.

PER SERVING: Calories: 409; Total Fat: 15g; Saturated Fat: 5g; Cholesterol: 50mg; Sodium: 292mg; Carbohydrates: 47g; Fiber: 17g; Added Sugars: 0g; Protein: 27g; Potassium: 1,466mg; Vitamin K: 90mcg

MUSHROOM BOLOGNESE

Store-bought pasta sauce is loaded with salt, but making your own is a cinch, and it freezes well. Use frozen chopped onion and garlic stir-in paste to make things easier. And if time is really tight, skip the mushrooms, tomato paste, and lentils. Even without them, this beats bottled sauce, which has more than 2 more teaspoons of salt than this recipe. Serve with pasta, roasted spaghetti squash, or sautéed zucchini noodles.

Serves 6 (1¼ cups per serving)

Hands-on time: 20 min

Total time: 30 min

1 pound extra-lean (7% fat) ground beef

½ teaspoon salt, divided (optional)

Freshly ground black pepper

1 onion, chopped

3 garlic cloves, minced

½ cup uncooked split red lentils, rinsed

1 (28-ounce) can whole, no-salt-added tomatoes

1 pound sliced mushrooms

⅔ cup water

2 tablespoons tomato paste

1 tablespoon dried oregano

1. Heat a large sauté pan over medium heat. When the pan is hot, add the beef and sprinkle with ¼ teaspoon salt (if using) and the pepper. Do not stir the meat until it is browned on the bottom, 2 to 3 minutes. Add the onion and garlic, and stir periodically until the beef is no longer pink, 5 to 7 minutes.

2. Turn up the heat and add the lentils, tomatoes with their juice, mushrooms, water, tomato paste, and oregano. When it boils, reduce the heat to medium and simmer, stirring occasionally, until the lentils are soft, about 15 minutes.

3. Taste, and add an extra ¼ teaspoon of salt and pepper, if desired.

SUBSTITUTION TIP: Simply skip the beef and double the lentils to make this a vegan entrée.

LEFTOVERS: Freeze the sauce in meal-size portions, about 1 cup per person. Thaw for 24 hours in the fridge or thaw in the microwave on 50 percent power for 5 to 15 minutes, depending on the quantity. Reheat on the stovetop.

PER SERVING: Calories: 225; Total Fat: 6g; Saturated Fat: 2g; Cholesterol: 48mg; Sodium: 266mg; Carbohydrates: 21g; Fiber: 5g; Added Sugars: 0g; Protein: 24g; Potassium: 947mg; Vitamin K: 8mcg

CHIPOTLE CHILI

Chili can be heavy, but this vegetable-rich version freshens it up with maple syrup to gently balance the spices. Use lean ground turkey, chicken, veal, or bison instead of beef, if you prefer. If you're in a hurry, use frozen onions and peppers instead of fresh. Top with sliced avocado, Fresh Tomato Salsa (page 182), scallions, jalapeños, fresh cilantro, hot sauce, shredded Cheddar cheese, Baked Tortilla Chips (page 155), plain yogurt, and/or sour cream.

Serves 6 (2 cups per serving)

Hands-on time: 20 min

Total time: 30 min

1 tablespoon canola or sunflower oil

2 onions, chopped

1 pound extra-lean (7% fat) ground beef

2 tablespoons chili powder

1 tablespoon Salt-Free Southwest Seasoning Mix (page 175) or Mrs. Dash, plus more if needed

½ teaspoon salt, divided

1 (28-ounce) can no-salt-added whole tomatoes

1 (5.5-ounce) can tomato paste

2 (15-ounce) cans no-salt-added beans of your choice, rinsed and drained

2 red bell peppers, seeded and chopped

2 medium zucchini, cut into bite-size pieces

1 tablespoon pure maple syrup

1. In a large pot, heat the oil. Add the beef and onions, and cook over medium-high heat, stirring to brown evenly, 7 to 10 minutes.

2. Add the chili powder, Southwest seasoning, and ¼ teaspoon of salt and stir for 1 minute. Add the tomatoes with their juice, tomato paste, beans, bell peppers, zucchini, and maple syrup. Turn up the heat to bring it to a boil, then turn it down to medium-low and simmer for 10 minutes.

3. Taste, and add another ¼ teaspoon of salt or more Southwest Seasoning, if desired.

SUBSTITUTION TIP: For a vegan version, just skip the meat. If the chili is too saucy for you, add more veggies—any kind you like.

PER SERVING: Calories: 347; Total Fat: 9g; Saturated Fat: 2g; Cholesterol: 48mg; Sodium: 365mg; Carbohydrates: 41g; Fiber: 14g; Added Sugars: 2g; Protein: 27g; Potassium: 1,473mg; Vitamin K: 12mcg

SOUTHWEST STEAK SKILLET

DASH

Thanks to my sister Tracy for sharing this favorite quick recipe. Like many of the meat recipes in this book, this dish features less meat than is typical, to make room for vegetables and plant-based protein foods like these black beans. Don't worry; there's plenty of protein. You can substitute another lean cut of beef, or boneless, skinless chicken breasts or thighs, if you prefer. Serve it with a light salad or fresh fruit.

Serves 4

Hands-on time: 25 min

Total time: 25 min

⅔ cup uncooked quinoa

1 tablespoon canola or sunflower oil

12 ounces top sirloin beef, trimmed and thinly sliced

½ red onion, chopped

1 green bell pepper, seeded and chopped

1 cup no-salt-added black beans, rinsed and drained

⅔ cup reduced-sodium chicken broth

1 tablespoon Salt-Free Southwest Seasoning Mix (page 175) or Mrs. Dash, plus more if needed

1 avocado, peeled, pitted, and diced

½ cup Fresh Tomato Salsa (page 182) or lower-sodium store-bought salsa

1. Cook the quinoa according to the package directions.

2. Meanwhile, heat the oil in a heavy skillet over medium-high heat. When it is hot, cook the steak slices until just cooked through, 3 to 4 minutes. Transfer to a plate.

3. Sauté the onion and pepper in the pan drippings until soft, 4 to 5 minutes. Turn the heat down to medium, if needed, to prevent them from burning. Add the black beans, broth, and Southwest seasoning. Turn the heat down to medium, cover, and cook, for 5 minutes.

4. Stir in the cooked quinoa when it is ready. Return the steak to the pan. Taste and add more Southwest Seasoning, if desired. Garnish with avocado and salsa.

FLAVOR BOOST: Add a squirt of hot sauce on top.

PER SERVING: Calories: 440; Total Fat: 22g; Saturated Fat: 5g; Cholesterol: 59mg; Sodium: 158mg; Carbohydrates: 36g; Fiber: 9g; Added Sugars: 0g; Protein: 26g; Potassium: 925mg; Vitamin K: 18mcg

SEARED STEAK AND BOK CHOY SALAD

DASH

This dish gets protein from cashews and quinoa as well as the steak, so you can use less meat than usual. You can also leave the meat out entirely and make this with Crispy Tofu (page 186) for a vegan alternative. Look for tamari (or reduced-sodium soy sauce) with no more than 600 mg of sodium per tablespoon.

Serves 4

Hands-on time: 30 min

Total time: 30 min

For the salad

1 cup uncooked quinoa

12 ounces top sirloin beef or strip steak, trimmed of visible fat

⅛ teaspoon kosher salt (optional)

Freshly ground black pepper (optional)

1 tablespoon canola or sunflower oil

3 to 4 heads baby bok choy *or* 1 large head bok choy, finely chopped

2 scallions, finely chopped

⅓ cup chopped unsalted roasted cashews

For the dressing

¼ cup extra-virgin olive oil

3 tablespoons rice vinegar

2 tablespoons reduced-sodium tamari

2 tablespoons sugar

1. Cook the quinoa according to the package directions. While it's cooking, put a medium bowl in the freezer. When the quinoa is done, take the bowl out and transfer the quinoa to the bowl to cool for a few minutes.

2. Meanwhile, pat the steak dry with a paper towel, then sprinkle it with salt and pepper (if using). Heat the oil in a large, heavy skillet over high heat. When it is very hot, add the steak. Brown for 5 to 6 minutes on each side, until just about done to your liking. Transfer to a cutting board and let it sit for 5 minutes, then cut it into thin slices.

3. To make the dressing, whisk together the oil, vinegar, tamari, and sugar in a large bowl. Add the bok choy, scallions, and quinoa. Toss well with the dressing.

4. Top with the steak and cashews.

PER SERVING: Calories: 526; Total Fat: 29g; Saturated Fat: 5g; Cholesterol: 58mg; Sodium: 500mg; Carbohydrates: 40g; Fiber: 5g; Added Sugars: 5g; Protein: 30g; Potassium: 1,055mg; Vitamin K: 105mcg

ALBERTA STEAK SALAD WITH ROASTED BABY POTATOES

DASH

My home province of Alberta, Canada, is known for beef. But we also grow some of the sweetest root vegetables around, thanks to warm days and frosty nights. This recipe features quintessential Alberta foods. Use what you have, improvise the rest, and enjoy.

Serves 4

Hands-on time: 30 min

Total time: 30 min

1½ pounds small new potatoes

2 tablespoons canola or sunflower oil, divided

½ teaspoon kosher salt, divided

Freshly ground black pepper

1 pound beef tenderloin steaks, trimmed of visible fat

1 head butter lettuce, torn into pieces

½ cup no-salt-added canned chickpeas, rinsed and drained

1 baby cucumber, sliced

1 medium carrot, peeled and shredded or spiralized

½ cup Red Wine Vinaigrette (page 178)

1 medium beet, peeled and shredded or spiralized

1. Preheat the oven to 400°F.

2. Spread the potatoes on a rimmed baking sheet. Add 1 tablespoon of oil, ¼ teaspoon of salt, and pepper. Toss well, and slide the baking sheet into the oven; roast the potatoes for 30 minutes.

3. Meanwhile, pat the steaks dry with a paper towel, and season with the remaining ¼ teaspoon of salt and pepper. Heat the remaining 1 tablespoon of oil in an oven-safe skillet over medium-high heat. When the skillet is very hot, cook the steaks until they are browned to your liking, 2 to 3 minutes per side. (Reduce the heat if the steaks are burning.) Put the skillet with the steaks in the oven, and roast to your desired level of doneness, 7 to 10 minutes. (A meat thermometer should read between 120°F for rare to 145°F for medium-well done. The temperature will continue to rise while the meat rests.)

4. While the meat and potatoes are cooking, combine the lettuce, chickpeas, cucumber, and carrot in a large bowl.

→

5. When the steak is ready, transfer it to a cutting board and tent with aluminum foil. Let it rest for at least 5 minutes before slicing against the grain.

6. Toss the salad with the vinaigrette, and top with the steak and beets. Serve the potatoes on the side.

COOKING TIP: If you don't have an oven-safe skillet, put a roasting pan in the oven to get hot, and transfer the steaks to the pan when it's time for them to go into the oven.

PER SERVING: Calories: 536; Total Fat: 28g; Saturated Fat: 5g; Cholesterol: 69mg; Sodium: 474mg; Carbohydrates: 42g; Fiber: 7g; Added Sugars: 1g; Protein: 31g; Potassium: 1,383mg; Vitamin K: 65mcg

SLICED PORK LOIN FOR SANDWICHES

Processed meat is convenient for sandwiches and wraps, but people who eat it frequently are more likely to get heart disease, diabetes, and some cancers. This simple alternative contains a fraction of the sodium and no nitrites. The key is to not overcook the pork. Use a meat thermometer, and take the pork out of the oven when the thickest part has reached 145°F. A hint of pink is fine. Make sure to let the meat rest for at least 5 minutes before slicing, to gently finish cooking.

Serves 4

Hands-on time: 10 min

Total time: 30 min

1 teaspoon onion powder

½ teaspoon garlic powder

½ teaspoon dried thyme

¼ teaspoon kosher salt

¼ teaspoon freshly ground black pepper

1 (1-pound) boneless pork tenderloin roast

1 tablespoon canola or sunflower oil

1. Preheat the oven to 425°F.

2. Mix the onion powder, garlic powder, thyme, salt, and pepper in a small bowl. Trim the tenderloin of any silverskin, and pat dry. Rub all over with the seasoning.

3. Heat the oil in a large, oven-safe skillet over medium-high heat. (If you don't have an oven-safe skillet, use a regular skillet and place an aluminum foil–lined roasting pan in the oven to heat up.) When the skillet is very hot, sear the pork for 2 minutes on each side. Transfer the skillet to the oven (or transfer the steak to the roasting pan).

4. Cook until the internal temperature reaches 145°F, about 15 minutes. Tent lightly with foil for at least 5 minutes before slicing.

FLAVOR BOOST: Season this however you like. Try the various salt-free seasoning blends, chili powder, Italian seasoning, curry powder, or Chinese five-spice blend.

PER SERVING: Calories: 158; Total Fat: 6g; Saturated Fat: 1g; Cholesterol: 74mg; Sodium: 181mg; Carbohydrates: 1g; Fiber: 0g; Added Sugars: 0g; Protein: 24g; Potassium: 464mg; Vitamin K: 5mcg

PORK CHOPS WITH MUSHROOM GRAVY

DASH

Think of this as a lighter version of the classic comfort food, pork chops with condensed cream of mushroom soup, only with more mushrooms and less salt. If you have a hungry crowd, serve this over Hearty Mashed Potatoes (page 69). Balance it with a green salad (there are several in chapter 3) instead of the spinach.

Serves 4

Hands-on time: 15 min

Total time: 15 min

1 recipe Mushroom and Thyme Gravy (page 185)

1 tablespoon canola or sunflower oil

4 bone-in pork loin chops

¼ teaspoon kosher salt

Freshly ground black pepper

1 (11-ounce) package baby spinach *or* 2 bunches spinach, torn into bite-size pieces

1. In a small saucepan, bring the gravy to a simmer over low heat.

2. Heat the oil in a large, heavy skillet over medium-high heat. Pat the pork chops dry, and season both sides with salt and pepper. When the oil is hot, add the pork chops and cook without touching for 3 to 4 minutes on each side, until the pork reaches an internal temperature of 145°F. The meat should be pale and white with mostly clear juices. Transfer the pork chops to a plate, and tent with aluminum foil.

3. Turn the heat down, and add the spinach and a splash of water to the pan. Cook for 1 to 2 minutes, until the spinach is wilted.

4. Serve the pork on a bed of spinach, topped with the gravy.

PER SERVING: Calories: 326; Total Fat: 20g; Saturated Fat: 5g; Cholesterol: 74mg; Sodium: 485mg; Carbohydrates: 10g; Fiber: 3g; Added Sugars: 0g; Protein: 27g; Potassium: 876mg; Vitamin K: 381mcg

MANGO AND PORK STIR-FRY

DASH

In this recipe, we freshen up a stir-fry with fruit. There are a lot of shortcuts to make this dish easier: Look for presliced pork in your supermarket. Use 2 cups frozen stir-fry vegetables in place of the bell pepper and snow peas. Use garlic powder and ground ginger instead of fresh. It's all good. Serve it over cooked barley, brown rice, or quinoa.

Serves 4

Hands-on time: 30 min

Total time: 30 min

1 (1-pound) boneless pork tenderloin

¼ teaspoon kosher salt (optional)

Freshly ground black pepper (optional)

⅓ cup sesame seeds

1 tablespoon canola or sunflower oil

2 teaspoons minced fresh ginger

2 garlic cloves, minced

1 red bell pepper, seeded and chopped

2 tablespoons rice vinegar

1½ tablespoons reduced-sodium tamari

2 teaspoons sesame oil

1 cup frozen mango chunks, any large pieces cut in half

1 cup snow peas, trimmed

1. Cut the tenderloin in half lengthwise, then thinly slice each half. Season with salt and pepper (if using).

2. Heat a large, heavy skillet over medium heat. When it's hot, add the sesame seeds and toast, stirring frequently, until lightly browned, 3 to 5 minutes. Immediately transfer them to a small bowl.

3. Add the oil to the skillet. When it's hot, add the pork. Sauté until lightly browned, 3 to 5 minutes. Add the ginger and garlic, and cook for a minute more. Transfer to a plate. Add the bell pepper to the skillet and cook for 3 to 4 minutes.

4. Add the rice vinegar, tamari, and sesame oil to the bowl with the sesame seeds, and whisk until mixed. Add the sauce and mango to the skillet. Cook until the mango is warm, about 2 minutes. Add the snow peas and pork, and cook until just warmed through.

FLAVOR BOOST: Add ½ teaspoon red pepper flakes or several thinly sliced scallions when you add the ginger and garlic.

PER SERVING: Calories: 306; Total Fat: 14g; Saturated Fat: 2g; Cholesterol: 74mg; Sodium: 451mg; Carbohydrates: 17g; Fiber: 5g; Added Sugars: 0g; Protein: 29g; Potassium: 726mg; Vitamin K: 15mcg

SWEET MOROCCAN PORK AND CARROTS

DASH

One of the quickest ways to serve lean pork tenderloin is to cut it cross-wise into medallions and pan-fry them. Baby carrots are convenient and nutritious, but they're not always the tastiest carrots. This sauce fixes that problem and jazzes up the pork, too.

Serves 4

Hands-on time: 25 min

Total time: 30 min

1 (1-pound) boneless pork tenderloin roast

¼ teaspoon kosher salt

Freshly ground black pepper

1 tablespoon canola or sunflower oil

1 large sweet onion, cut into wedges

1 cup reduced-sodium chicken broth

1 pound baby carrots

2 tablespoons honey

¼ teaspoon ground ginger

¼ teaspoon ground cinnamon

¼ teaspoon ground cumin

¼ teaspoon ground turmeric

1 cup uncooked whole-wheat couscous

1 teaspoon freshly squeezed lemon juice

1. Trim the tenderloin of any silverskin, and pat it dry. Slice the tenderloin into ½-inch-thick medallions. Season with salt and pepper.

2. Heat the oil in a large skillet over medium-high heat. When the oil is very hot, cook the pork until it is browned on both sides, about 3 minutes per side. Transfer to a plate, and tent with aluminum foil.

3. Turn the heat down to medium, and sauté the onion until softened, 3 to 4 minutes. Turn it up to high, and add the chicken broth and carrots, then the honey, ginger, cinnamon, cumin, and turmeric. When the broth is boiling vigorously, turn the heat back to medium and cook until the carrots are tender, 7 to 8 minutes.

4. Meanwhile, cook the couscous according to the package directions.

5. Return the pork to the skillet, along with the lemon juice, and cook until everything is just heated through. Serve the pork and vegetables over the couscous.

PER SERVING: Calories: 426; Total Fat: 7g; Saturated Fat: 1g; Cholesterol: 83mg; Sodium: 347mg; Carbohydrates: 55g; Fiber: 6g; Added Sugars: 9g; Protein: 35g; Potassium: 997mg; Vitamin K: 13mcg

PAN-SEARED PORK MEDALLIONS WITH PEARS

DASH

Pair this dish with roasted vegetables or a light green salad for a satisfying weeknight dinner. For a little something extra, replace ½ cup of the chicken broth with ½ cup dry white wine.

Serves 4

Hands-on time: 25 min

Total time: 30 min

2 cups water

1 cup uncooked
pearl barley

1 (1-pound) boneless pork
tenderloin roast

½ teaspoon kosher salt

Freshly ground
black pepper

1 tablespoon canola or
sunflower oil

3 celery stalks, chopped

2 shallots, chopped

1 garlic clove, minced

1 tablespoon
unsalted butter

½ teaspoon dried rosemary

¼ teaspoon ground ginger

1 tablespoon
all-purpose flour

1 cup reduced-sodium
chicken broth

1 (15-ounce) can sliced
pears, drained

1. Bring the water to a boil in a large pot over high heat. Add the barley. Cover the pot, reduce the heat, and simmer for 25 minutes or until tender.

2. Meanwhile, trim the tenderloin of any silverskin, and pat it dry. Slice the tenderloin into ½-inch-thick medallions. Sprinkle with salt and pepper.

3. Heat the oil in a large skillet over medium-high heat. When it is hot, cook the pork until it is browned on both sides, about 3 minutes per side. Transfer to a plate, and tent with aluminum foil.

4. Add the celery, shallots, garlic, butter, rosemary, and ginger to the skillet, and sauté for 2 to 3 minutes. Stir in the flour until blended. Then gradually add the broth, stirring constantly, until the mixture comes to a boil. Cook and stir for 1 minute, until thickened.

5. Add the pears, and return the pork to the skillet. Taste and adjust the seasoning, if needed. Serve the pork, pears, and sauce over the barley.

PER SERVING: Calories: 438; Total Fat: 10g; Saturated Fat: 3g; Cholesterol: 82mg; Sodium: 362mg; Carbohydrates: 58g; Fiber: 10g; Added Sugars: 0g; Protein: 30g; Potassium: 868mg; Vitamin K: 13mcg

RED BEANS, SAUSAGE, AND RICE

DASH

Here's a lighter, vegetable-rich version of classic rice and beans. If you can't find andouille, substitute bratwurst or kielbasa. Look for a brand with less than 700 mg sodium per 3-ounce serving. You can cook the rice with the rest of the dish, adding it and the water when you add the tomatoes.

Serves 4

Hands-on time: 20 min

Total time: 30 min

¾ cup uncooked parboiled brown rice *or* 2 cups cooked brown rice

1 tablespoon canola or sunflower oil

6 ounces smoked andouille sausage, cut into bite-size pieces

1 onion, chopped

1 green bell pepper, seeded and chopped

1 red bell pepper, seeded and chopped

4 garlic cloves, minced

1 (28-ounce) can no-salt-added whole tomatoes

1 (15-ounce) can no-salt-added kidney beans, rinsed and drained

1 teaspoon ground cumin

1 teaspoon dried thyme

½ teaspoon red pepper flakes

¼ teaspoon freshly ground black pepper

1. Start the rice cooking according to the package directions.

2. Meanwhile, heat the oil in a large, heavy skillet over medium-high heat. Add the sausage and cook until lightly browned, 3 to 4 minutes. Add the onion, bell peppers, and garlic, and cook until softened, 5 to 6 minutes.

3. Stir in the tomatoes with their juice, beans, cumin, thyme, red pepper flakes, and black pepper. Bring to a boil. Add the rice whether it's ready or not (including any water yet to be absorbed). Turn the heat down to medium-low, and cover. Simmer until the rice is fully cooked, 5 to 10 minutes.

4. Taste, and adjust the seasonings.

INGREDIENT TIP: Andouille is a smoked pork sausage that originated in France and is used in Louisiana Creole cuisine. Find it where you buy bacon and hot dogs. The amount of sausage in this dish is minimal—just enough to provide a rich flavor to the beans and vegetables.

PER SERVING: Calories: 395; Total Fat: 11g; Saturated Fat: 3g; Cholesterol: 26mg; Sodium: 337mg; Carbohydrates: 58g; Fiber: 15g; Added Sugars: 0g; Protein: 20g; Potassium: 1,001mg; Vitamin K: 17mcg

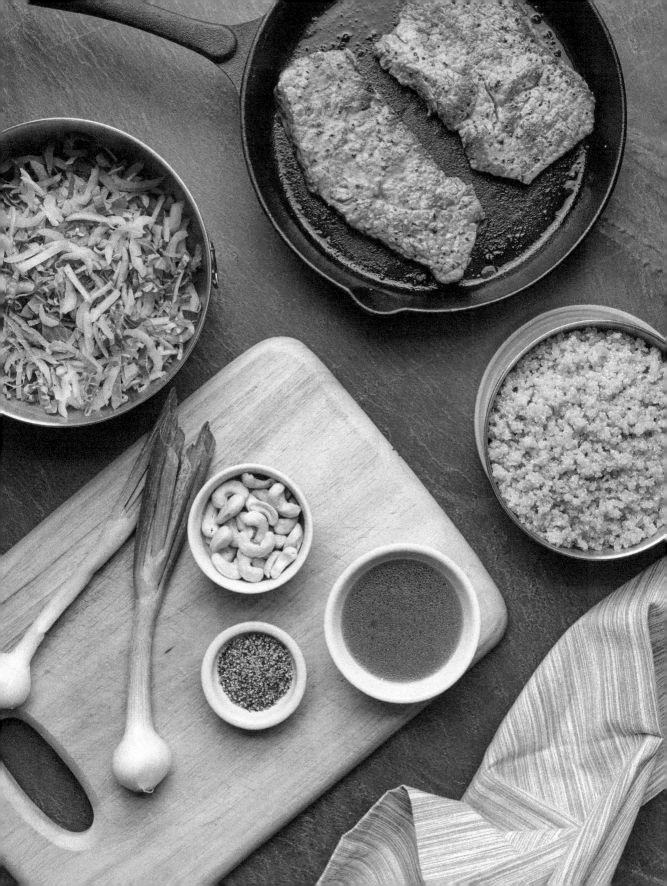

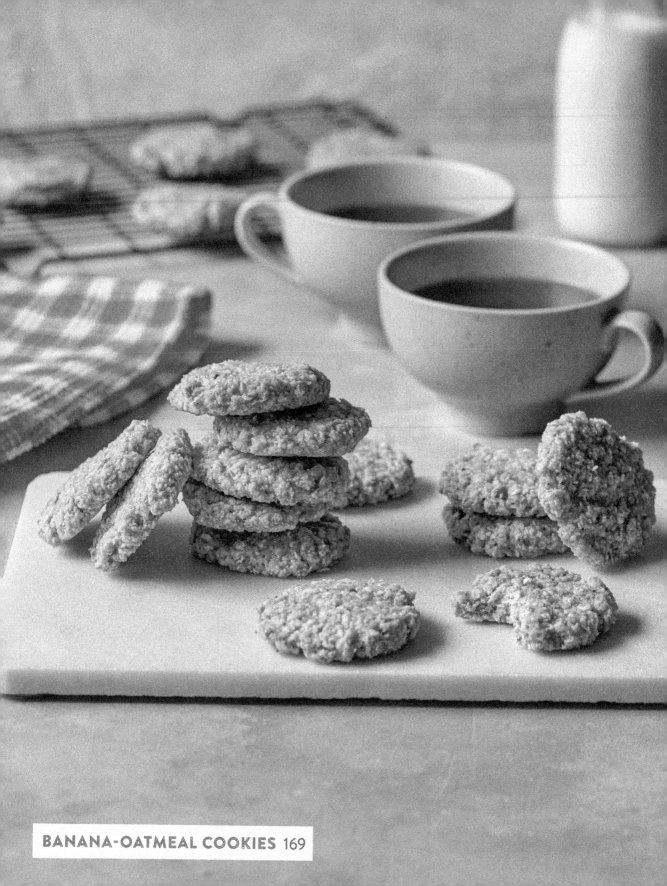

BANANA-OATMEAL COOKIES 169

SNACKS AND SWEET TREATS

SESAME-GARLIC EDAMAME

DASH • MEDITERRANEAN • VEGAN • PORTABLE

Edamame is the Japanese word for young soybeans. You may have had them as an appetizer at a Japanese restaurant, but now this fiber- and protein-rich food is commonly available frozen, both shelled and not. The typical way to season them is with salt or soy sauce, but you can lighten up on those if you boost the flavors in other ways, as in this version.

Serves 4

Hands-on time: 10 min

Total time: 10 min

1 (14-ounce) package frozen edamame in their shells

1 tablespoon canola or sunflower oil

1 tablespoon toasted sesame oil

3 garlic cloves, minced

½ teaspoon kosher salt

¼ teaspoon red pepper flakes (or more)

1. Bring a large pot of water to a boil over high heat. Add the edamame, and cook just long enough to warm them up, 2 to 3 minutes.

2. Meanwhile, heat the canola oil, sesame oil, garlic, salt, and red pepper flakes in a large skillet over medium heat for 1 to 2 minutes, then remove the pan from the heat.

3. Drain the edamame and add them to the skillet, tossing to combine.

INGREDIENT TIP: The idea is to eat the beans, not the pods, as my husband learned the hard way on one of our first dates. Just pinch the pods with your thumb and index finger, and the beans will pop out straight into your mouth.

PER SERVING: Calories: 173; Total Fat: 12g; Saturated Fat: 1g; Cholesterol: 0mg; Sodium: 246mg; Carbohydrates: 8g; Fiber: 5g; Added Sugars: 0g; Protein: 11g; Potassium: 487mg; Vitamin K: 34mcg

152   30-MINUTE HEART HEALTHY COOKBOOK

ROSEMARY AND WHITE BEAN DIP

DASH • MEDITERRANEAN • VEGAN • NO-COOK • PORTABLE

Hummus is great, but did you know you can make similar dips with other legumes and flavors? This recipe has about half the sodium of commercial hummus, so if you want more flavor, try adding more of the other ingredients first, and then add a touch more salt if needed. Dig in with your favorite raw vegetables, crackers, or Baked Tortilla Chips (page 155).

Serves 10 (¼ cup per serving)

Hands-on time: 10 min

Total time: 10 min

1 (15-ounce) can cannellini beans, rinsed and drained

2 tablespoons extra-virgin olive oil

1 garlic clove, peeled

1 teaspoon finely chopped fresh rosemary

Pinch cayenne pepper

Freshly ground black pepper

1 (7.5-ounce) jar marinated artichoke hearts, drained

1. Blend the beans, oil, garlic, rosemary, cayenne pepper, and black pepper in a food processor until smooth.

2. Add the artichoke hearts, and pulse until roughly chopped but not puréed.

SUBSTITUTION TIP: Great northern or navy beans work fine for this, too.

PER SERVING: Calories: 75; Total Fat: 5g; Saturated Fat: 1g; Cholesterol: 0mg; Sodium: 139mg; Carbohydrates: 6g; Fiber: 3g; Added Sugars: 0g; Protein: 2g; Potassium: 75mg; Vitamin K: 1mcg

GARLICKY KALE CHIPS

DASH • MEDITERRANEAN • VEGAN • 5-INGREDIENT • PORTABLE

Kale chips are surprisingly good, winning over even the most stubborn kale skeptics. The trick is to cook them long enough that they're crispy, but not so long that they turn to dust. You can do these faster at a higher temperature, but then the window between perfect and overdone will be very short. Every oven is different, so watch closely during the last few minutes of cooking.

Serves 4

Hands-on time: 5 min

Total time: 25 min

1 bunch curly kale

2 teaspoons extra-virgin olive oil

¼ teaspoon kosher salt

¼ teaspoon garlic powder (optional)

1. Preheat the oven to 325°F. Line a rimmed baking sheet with parchment paper.

2. Remove the tough stems from the kale, and tear the leaves into squares about the size of big potato chips (they'll shrink when cooked).

3. Transfer the kale to a large bowl, and drizzle with the oil. Massage with your fingers for 1 to 2 minutes to coat well. Spread out on the baking sheet.

4. Cook for 8 minutes, then toss and cook for another 7 minutes and check them. Take them out as soon as they feel crispy, likely within the next 5 minutes.

5. Sprinkle with salt and garlic powder (if using). Enjoy immediately.

FLAVOR BOOST: Instead of garlic powder, try ground cumin, onion powder, cayenne pepper, Parmesan cheese, flavored olive oil, or a salt-free seasoning mix.

COOKING TIP: The kale has to be very dry to get crispy. If possible, wash and dry it earlier in the day and leave it on a kitchen towel. Otherwise, use a salad spinner and/ or paper towel to remove as much moisture as possible.

PER SERVING: Calories: 28; Total Fat: 2g; Saturated Fat: 0g; Cholesterol: 0mg; Sodium: 126mg; Carbohydrates: 2g; Fiber: 1g; Added Sugars: 0g; Protein: 1g; Potassium: 81mg; Vitamin K: 114mcg

BAKED TORTILLA CHIPS

DASH • MEDITERRANEAN • VEGAN • 5-INGREDIENT • PORTABLE

Baked tortilla chips are crispy and delicious, especially fresh out of the oven. These are so much tastier than store-bought baked chips, and you can make them with whole-grain tortillas. They're also good made with corn tortillas or small pitas.

Serves 4

Hands-on time: 5 min

Total time: 20 min

1 tablespoon canola or sunflower oil

4 medium whole-wheat tortillas

⅛ teaspoon coarse salt

1. Preheat the oven to 350°F.

2. Brush the oil onto both sides of each tortilla. Stack them on a large cutting board, and cut the entire stack at once, cutting the stack into 8 wedges of each tortilla. Transfer the tortilla pieces to a rimmed baking sheet. Sprinkle a little salt over each chip.

3. Bake for 10 minutes, and then flip the chips. Bake for another 3 to 5 minutes, until they're just starting to brown.

FLAVOR BOOST: Mix the salt with ½ teaspoon each ground cumin and chili powder before sprinkling it onto the chips. Watch that you don't overcook, because they'll look brown from the start.

PER SERVING: Calories: 194; Total Fat: 11g; Saturated Fat: 2g; Cholesterol: 0mg; Sodium: 347mg; Carbohydrates: 20g; Fiber: 4g; Added Sugars: 0g; Protein: 4g; Potassium: 111mg; Vitamin K: 7mcg

SPICY GUACAMOLE

MEDITERRANEAN • VEGAN • NO-COOK • PORTABLE

There are many variations on guacamole, and this combination is bursting with flavor. Avocados are high in fiber, healthy fats, and vitamin E. They make an excellent replacement for mayonnaise or cheese in many dishes. If you have a mini-chopper, use it to mince the jalapeño, red onion, cilantro, and garlic for you. If time is tight, just mash an avocado and mix it with lime juice and salt.

Serves 4 (about 3 tablespoons per serving)

Hands-on time: 15 min

Total time: 15 min

1 ripe avocado, peeled, pitted, and mashed

1½ tablespoons freshly squeezed lime juice

1 tablespoon minced jalapeño pepper, or to taste

1 tablespoon minced red onion

1 tablespoon chopped fresh cilantro

1 garlic clove, minced

⅛ to ¼ teaspoon kosher salt

Freshly ground black pepper

Combine the avocado, lime juice, jalapeño, onion, cilantro, garlic, salt, and pepper in a large bowl, and mix well.

FLAVOR BOOST: Add ½ teaspoon ground cumin or chili powder for another flavor dimension.

INGREDIENT TIP: Keep avocados in the fridge until a day or two before needed, then ripen them on the countertop.

PER SERVING: Calories: 61; Total Fat: 5g; Saturated Fat: 1g; Cholesterol: 0mg; Sodium: 123mg; Carbohydrates: 4g; Fiber: 2g; Added Sugars: 0g; Protein: 1g; Potassium: 195mg; Vitamin K: 8mcg

CHICKPEA FATTEH

DASH • MEDITERRANEAN • VEGETARIAN

Thanks to my Lebanese friends, Nariman and Cristel, for introducing me to this delicious appetizer. It's a delight for guests—and a great way to use up stale pita bread. Pine nuts are traditional but pricey, so feel free to substitute slivered almonds. Pomegranate isn't traditional, but it's a pretty addition.

Serves 8

Hands-on time: 25 min

Total time: 25 min

2 (4-inch) whole-wheat pitas

4 tablespoons extra-virgin olive oil, divided

1 (15-ounce) can no-salt-added chickpeas, rinsed and drained

⅓ cup pine nuts

1 cup plain 1% yogurt

2 garlic cloves, minced

¼ teaspoon salt

½ cup pomegranate seeds (optional)

1. Preheat the oven to 375°F.

2. Cut the pitas into 1-inch squares (no need to separate the two halves), and toss with 2 tablespoons of oil in a large bowl. Spread onto a rimmed baking sheet and bake, shaking the sheet occasionally, until golden brown, about 10 minutes.

3. Meanwhile, gently warm the chickpeas and 1 tablespoon of oil in a small saucepan over medium-low heat, 4 to 5 minutes.

4. Toast the pine nuts in a skillet with the remaining 1 tablespoon of oil over medium heat until golden brown, 4 to 5 minutes.

5. Mix the yogurt with the garlic and salt in a small bowl.

6. Transfer the toasted pitas to a wide serving bowl. Top with the chickpeas. Drizzle with the yogurt mixture, then top with the pine nuts and pomegranate seeds (if using).

SUBSTITUTION TIP: If you use Greek yogurt, thin it out with 2 tablespoons of water.

PER SERVING: Calories: 198; Total Fat: 12g; Saturated Fat: 2g; Cholesterol: 2mg; Sodium: 144mg; Carbohydrates: 18g; Fiber: 3g; Added Sugars: 0g; Protein: 6g; Potassium: 236mg; Vitamin K: 9mcg

MARINATED BERRIES

DASH • MEDITERRANEAN • VEGAN • NO-COOK

Balsamic vinegar and pepper seem like strange partners for berries, but it works! Enjoy these on their own or as a topping for spinach salad or plain Greek yogurt sweetened with honey. You'll be one delicious step closer to the 8 to 10 servings a day of fruit and vegetables in the blood-pressure-friendly DASH eating pattern.

Serves 4

Hands-on time: 5 min

Total time: 30 min

2 cups fresh strawberries, hulled and quartered

1 cup fresh blueberries (optional)

2 tablespoons sugar

1 tablespoon balsamic vinegar

2 tablespoons chopped fresh mint (optional)

⅛ teaspoon freshly ground black pepper

1. Gently toss the strawberries, blueberries (if using), sugar, vinegar, mint (if using), and pepper in a large nonreactive bowl.

2. Let the flavors blend together for at least 25 minutes, or as long as 2 hours.

INGREDIENT TIP: This recipe works best with a good balsamic vinegar. Look for the terms *"D.O.P.," "Condimento,"* or *"IGP"* on the bottle.

PER SERVING: Calories: 73; Total Fat: 8g; Saturated Fat: 8g; Cholesterol: 0mg; Sodium: 4mg; Carbohydrates: 18g; Fiber: 2g; Added Sugars: 6g; Protein: 1g; Potassium: 162mg; Vitamin K: 9mcg

PUMPKIN-TURMERIC LATTE

DASH • VEGETARIAN • PORTABLE

If you love flavored coffee drinks but feel guilty about them, don't. You can make a reasonable facsimile of most coffee drinks at home with less sugar, and milk gives you protein and blood pressure–friendly minerals like calcium and potassium. Make sure you get plain pumpkin purée, not the pumpkin pie filling that has added spices and sugar. For a vegan version, use a plant-based milk.

Serves 1

Hands-on time: 10 min

Total time: 10 min

½ cup brewed espresso *or* 1 cup brewed strong coffee

¼ cup canned pumpkin purée

1 teaspoon vanilla extract

1 teaspoon sugar

½ teaspoon ground turmeric

½ teaspoon ground cinnamon, plus more if needed

1 cup 1% milk

1. Combine the espresso, pumpkin, vanilla, sugar, turmeric, and cinnamon in a medium saucepan over medium heat, whisking occasionally.

2. Warm the milk over low heat in a small pan. When it is warm (not hot), whisk it vigorously (or mix with a blender or handheld frother) to make it foamy.

3. Pour the hot coffee mixture into a mug, then top with the frothy milk. Sprinkle with more cinnamon, if desired.

INGREDIENT TIP: Some studies suggest that pumpkin, turmeric, and cinnamon, like other plant-based foods, may help fight disease in various ways, such as reducing inflammation and helping control blood sugar. Although our understanding of their actions is far from conclusive, it's safe to say that using spices and vegetables to flavor drinks beats sugary syrups.

COOKING TIP: You can also heat the milk in the microwave in a mason jar without the lid. When the milk is warm, put the lid on and shake vigorously. Or just warm it up with the coffee. You won't have the foam, but you will have all the flavor.

PER SERVING: Calories: 169; Total Fat: 3g; Saturated Fat: 2g; Cholesterol: 12mg; Sodium: 128mg; Carbohydrates: 26g; Fiber: 3g; Added Sugars: 5g; Protein: 9g; Potassium: 665mg; Vitamin K: 11mcg

DARK HOT CHOCOLATE

VEGAN • 5-INGREDIENT • ONE POT • PORTABLE

This drink is creamy and smooth, thanks to vanilla soy milk and real chocolate, but it has less than half the sugar of typical hot cocoa. For a warm morning jump-start, add this to your coffee for a homemade mocha. You can make this with dairy milk, but you'll need to at least double the chocolate for it to taste good. Try vanilla almond milk if you don't drink soy milk.

Serves 2

Hands-on time: 5 min

Total time: 5 min

1¾ cups vanilla soy milk

1 ounce dark chocolate
(70% cacao or more),
broken into small pieces

1. Heat the soy milk in a small saucepan over medium-high heat and add the chocolate. When the milk starts bubbling, turn the heat to low.

2. Whisk until the chocolate is melted and fully incorporated. Tip the pot to make sure there is no remaining chocolate on the bottom.

INGREDIENT TIP: Dark chocolate typically comes in 3.5-ounce bars. Use about a quarter of a bar.

PER SERVING: Calories: 149; Total Fat: 8g; Saturated Fat: 3g; Cholesterol: 0mg; Sodium: 105mg; Carbohydrates: 14g; Fiber: 2g; Added Sugars: 5g; Protein: 6g; Potassium: 351mg; Vitamin K: 4mcg

DARK CHOCOLATE AND CHERRY TRAIL MIX

DASH • MEDITERRANEAN • VEGAN • 5-INGREDIENT • NO-COOK • PORTABLE

It might seem odd to have a recipe for this, but packaged trail mix is heavy on cheap candy and dried fruit and light on nuts, which have been consistently connected to improved cardiac outcomes. This ratio is comparable to the calories in a granola bar, but with more fiber, healthy fat, and protein. Substitute whatever mix-ins you like or find on sale. Use coconut flakes and chopped dried mango or pineapple in place of the chocolate chips and dried cherries, for a tropical twist. Keep a small stash in your car, travel bag, or desk, with the rest of it in the freezer for freshness. (If it's hot out, leave out the chocolate, as it will melt.)

Makes 3 cups (¼ cup per serving)

Hands-on time: 5 min

Total time: 5 min

1 cup unsalted almonds

⅔ cup dried cherries

½ cup walnuts

½ cup sweet cinnamon-roasted chickpeas

¼ cup dark chocolate chips

1. Combine the almonds, cherries, walnuts, chickpeas, and chocolate chips in an airtight container.

2. Store at room temperature for up to 1 week or in the freezer for up to 3 months.

INGREDIENT TIP: The roasted chickpeas add fiber. Look for them where you buy nuts and seeds. If you can't find sweet cinnamon, substitute another sweet flavor or soy nuts, or leave them out.

PER SERVING: Calories: 174; Total Fat: 12g; Saturated Fat: 2g; Cholesterol: 0mg; Sodium: 18mg; Carbohydrates: 16g; Fiber: 4g; Added Sugars: 7g; Protein: 5g; Potassium: 134mg; Vitamin K: 0mcg

HAPPY HEART ENERGY BITES

These little nuggets are an easy, satisfying way to keep you fueled on the go. Compare them to a typical granola bar, and you'll find more fiber and protein. In addition, walnuts have omega-3 fat, and oats and ground flax give you cholesterol-lowering soluble fiber. Use smooth or chunky peanut butter, and substitute other nuts, seeds, and dried fruit for the walnuts and cranberries, to your taste.

Makes 30 (2 balls per serving)

Hands-on time: 20 min

Total time: 30 min

1 cup rolled oats

¾ cup chopped walnuts

½ cup natural peanut butter

½ cup ground flaxseed

¼ cup honey

¼ cup dried cranberries

1. Combine the oats, walnuts, peanut butter, flaxseed, honey, and cranberries in a large bowl. Refrigerate for 10 to 20 minutes, if you can, to make them easier to roll.

2. Roll into ¾-inch balls. Store in the fridge or freezer, if they don't disappear first.

SUBSTITUTION TIP: Make these vegan by using pure maple syrup instead of honey.

PER SERVING: Calories: 174; Total Fat: 10g; Saturated Fat: 1g; Cholesterol: 0mg; Sodium: 43mg; Carbohydrates: 17g; Fiber: 3g; Added Sugars: 7g; Protein: 5g; Potassium: 169mg; Vitamin K: 1mcg

CHOCOLATE-CASHEW SPREAD

DASH • MEDITERRANEAN • VEGETARIAN • NO-COOK • PORTABLE

Store-bought chocolate spread is mostly sugar and palm oil. Turns out you can make your own with heart-healthy cashews instead! Measure the oil first and then a teaspoon of honey into the same measuring spoon, so it doesn't stick. Taste it, and if you prefer more sweetness, add another teaspoon of honey. This works as a dip for bananas, raspberries, or pears, or as a spread on light rye crackers or sprouted-grain toast. Add another tablespoon of water if it's too thick for dipping fruit.

Makes ½ cup (2 tablespoons per serving)

Hands-on time: 10 min

Total time: 10 min

¼ cup unsalted cashew butter

3 tablespoons water

1½ tablespoons unsweetened cocoa powder

2 teaspoons honey

1 teaspoon extra-virgin olive oil

½ teaspoon vanilla extract

Pinch of ground cinnamon

Pinch of salt

Stir together the cashew butter, water, cocoa powder, honey, olive oil, vanilla, cinnamon, and salt in a large bowl until smooth, 2 to 3 minutes.

INGREDIENT TIP: You can make this with almond or peanut butter, but it will taste less like chocolate and more like almonds or peanuts. Cashew butter is smooth and has a neutral taste, which lets the chocolate sing. Look for it in the natural foods section of a well-stocked grocery store.

COOKING TIP: If any natural butter sits too long, it separates and the bottom gets quite thick. Add a little canola or sunflower oil, and give it a good stir. This spread is best very smooth, so if your cashew butter has hardened, blend it in a food processor or electric mixer.

SUBSTITUTION TIP: Substitute pure maple syrup for the honey to make a vegan spread.

PER SERVING: Calories: 108; Total Fat: 9g; Saturated Fat: 2g; Cholesterol: 0mg; Sodium: 93mg; Carbohydrates: 8g; Fiber: 1g; Added Sugars: 3g; Protein: 2g; Potassium: 92mg; Vitamin K: 5mcg

ALMOND BUTTER AND BANANA WRAP

DASH • VEGAN • 5-INGREDIENT • NO-COOK • PORTABLE

If you're heading out the door and suddenly realize you'll need something to eat before you get back, this is one of your fastest homemade grab-and-go options. It's great when you're on the move because it doesn't have to be refrigerated or heated, and it's a satisfying, nutritious alternative to fast food, packing healthy fats, protein, potassium, and fiber. Peanut butter and cashew butter work for this, too; if you need a nut-free option, try sunflower seed butter.

Serves 1

Hands-on time: 5 min

Total time: 5 min

2 tablespoons natural almond butter

1 whole-wheat tortilla

1 banana

1. Spread the almond butter on the tortilla.
2. Place the banana across the middle of the tortilla, and wrap it up. Cut into three pieces, if you like.

FLAVOR BOOST: Add a tablespoon of dried cranberries for sweetness, chopped walnuts for crunchy omega-3 fats, and/or hemp seeds for extra protein.

PER SERVING: Calories: 433; Total Fat: 22g; Saturated Fat: 4g; Cholesterol: 0mg; Sodium: 361mg; Carbohydrates: 52g; Fiber: 11g; Added Sugars: 0g; Protein: 12g; Potassium: 773mg; Vitamin K: 3mcg

MANGO CHILLER

Fruit for dessert doesn't have to be boring! This treat has a fresh, creamy taste with far less sugar than similar items you buy in the store, and a little protein and fiber for good measure. This looks pretty topped with fresh raspberries. Add a splash of coconut milk instead of dairy milk for a tropical twist. Soy or almond milk will also work.

Serves 4 (½ cup per serving)

Hands-on time: 5 min

Total time: 5 min

2 cups frozen mango chunks

½ cup plain 2% Greek yogurt

¼ cup 1% milk

2 teaspoons honey (optional)

1. Mix the mango and yogurt in a food processor or blender. Add the milk, a bit at a time, to get it to the consistency of soft ice cream.

2. Taste, and add honey if you like. Enjoy immediately.

FLAVOR BOOST: This also works with frozen bananas! They're so creamy you don't need anything but the banana—not even the yogurt and milk. But mix in a little peanut butter, honey, cocoa powder, chopped strawberry, or chocolate chips for fun.

PER SERVING: Calories: 85; Total Fat: 1g; Saturated Fat: 1g; Cholesterol: 4mg; Sodium: 17mg; Carbohydrates: 16g; Fiber: 1g; Added Sugars: 3g; Protein: 4g; Potassium: 197mg; Vitamin K: 3mcg

BLUEBERRY-RICOTTA SWIRL

DASH • VEGETARIAN • 5-INGREDIENT • ONE POT • PORTABLE

This is a quick, satisfying treat reminiscent of cheesecake. There are lots of fun variations: Instead of blueberries and lemon, try raspberries and grated chocolate, or pumpkin purée with a dash of cinnamon. This is a perfect use for Blueberry-Chia Jam (page 184), or make it with ½ teaspoon unsweetened cocoa powder and a few chocolate chips.

Serves 2

Hands-on time: 5 min

Total time: 5 min

½ cup fresh or frozen blueberries

½ cup part-skim ricotta cheese

1 teaspoon sugar

½ teaspoon lemon zest (optional)

1. If using frozen blueberries, warm them in a saucepan over medium heat until they are thawed but not hot.

2. Meanwhile, mix the sugar with the ricotta in a medium bowl.

3. Mix the blueberries into the ricotta, leaving a few out. Taste, and add more sugar if desired. Top with the remaining blueberries and lemon zest (if using).

COOKING TIP: Defrost the blueberries for about 15 seconds in the microwave if you prefer.

PER SERVING: Calories: 113; Total Fat: 5g; Saturated Fat: 3g; Cholesterol: 19mg; Sodium: 62mg; Carbohydrates: 10g; Fiber: 1g; Added Sugars: 2g; Protein: 7g; Potassium: 98mg; Vitamin K: 7mcg

STOVETOP APPLE CRISP

DASH • VEGETARIAN • PORTABLE

Apple crisp is always a pretty heart-healthy dessert—thanks to the fruit, the whole-grain oats, and the potential to top it with crunchy walnuts or pumpkin seeds. But for a weeknight (and sometimes breakfast) comfort food, try this quicker, lighter version of the classic. Or you can just cook the apples to go with oatmeal, if you don't have time for the crunchy topping.

Serves 4

Hands-on time: 15 min

Total time: 20 min

1 pound red apples, cored and sliced (about 5)

⅓ cup water

1 teaspoon plus 1 tablespoon packed brown sugar, divided

¼ teaspoon freshly squeezed lemon juice (optional)

¼ cup rolled oats

¼ cup chopped walnuts

1 tablespoon unsalted butter

¼ teaspoon ground cinnamon

Pinch salt

2 tablespoons dried cranberries (optional)

1. Put the apples and water in a large pot or sauté pan, and bring to a boil over medium-high heat. When the water starts to boil, turn the heat down to medium-low, cover, and cook for 5 to 10 minutes. Check it and stir every few minutes, adding more water if needed.

2. When the apples are just about soft enough for your liking, take the lid off and cook until any excess liquid has evaporated. Taste an apple; add 1 teaspoon of brown sugar if they're too tart, or add the lemon juice if they're too sweet. (The cooking time and additions needed will vary by type of apple and personal preference.)

→

3. Meanwhile, combine the oats, walnuts, butter, cinnamon, salt, and 1 tablespoon of brown sugar in a small skillet. Cook over medium heat, stirring occasionally, until everything is toasty and fragrant.

4. Top the stewed apples with the crispy nuts and oats, as well as a sprinkle of dried cranberries, if you like.

COOKING TIP: If you like this dish, an inexpensive apple slicer is a helpful tool, cutting the apple prep time down to about 1 minute. Also, you can cook the apples in the microwave in a microwave-safe bowl topped with a lid or plate. Add just 1 tablespoon of water. It should take about 5 minutes, depending on the type of apple and the power of your microwave.

PER SERVING: Calories: 185; Total Fat: 8g; Saturated Fat: 2g; Cholesterol: 8mg; Sodium: 42mg; Carbohydrates: 29g; Fiber: 4g; Added Sugars: 4g; Protein: 2g; Potassium: 182mg; Vitamin K: 3mcg

BANANA-OATMEAL COOKIES

VEGETARIAN • PORTABLE

If you feel that you must serve cookies when people visit, here are some that taste great and have two ingredients that support heart health—oats and bananas. In fact, don't wait for guests; make some just for you. If you don't want to eat them all, the crew at your local fire station would probably be happy to help you out.

Makes 30 medium cookies (1 per serving)

Hands-on time: 15 min

Total time: 30 min

½ cup Better Butter (page 176) *or* ¼ cup unsalted butter plus ¼ cup canola or sunflower oil

1 cup packed brown sugar

1 large egg

2 large, ripe bananas, mashed

2 teaspoons vanilla extract

½ cup all-purpose flour

½ cup whole-wheat flour

1 teaspoon salt

½ teaspoon baking soda

3 cups rolled oats

1. Preheat the oven to 375°F. Lightly oil two rimmed baking sheets.

2. Cream the Better Butter, brown sugar, and egg in a large bowl. Stir in the mashed bananas and vanilla.

3. In another medium bowl, combine the flours, salt, and baking soda. Add to the banana mixture. Mix in the oats.

4. Drop tablespoon-size rounds onto the baking sheets. Bake for 12 to 13 minutes, watching closely near the end so the cookies don't burn.

COOKING TIP: If your butter is hard, grate it into the bowl and it will soften up in no time.

PER SERVING: Calories: 118; Total Fat: 4g; Saturated Fat: 1g; Cholesterol: 10mg; Sodium: 104mg; Carbohydrates: 18g; Fiber: 2g; Added Sugars: 7g; Protein: 2g; Potassium: 78mg; Vitamin K: 2mcg

GRANO DOLCE LIGHT (SWEET WHEAT)

DASH • MEDITERRANEAN • VEGETARIAN

This is a simpler, lighter version of a delightfully nutritious traditional Italian dessert. Even so, it's quite substantial, so pair it for dinner with a light salad and perhaps a piece of grilled meat, fish, or chicken. Don't be afraid of the pomegranate; I've given simple seeding instructions in the tip. Or just use 1½ cups frozen pomegranate seeds.

Serves 6

Hands-on time: 20 min

Total time: 30 min

⅔ cup uncooked farro

⅛ teaspoon salt

¼ cup walnuts

¼ cup almonds

1 pomegranate

2 tablespoons plus 1 teaspoon honey, divided

½ cup 5% plain Greek yogurt

1 teaspoon apple cider vinegar

¼ teaspoon ground cinnamon

2 ounces dark chocolate (70%+ cacao), cut into ½-inch squares

1. Preheat the oven to 350°F.

2. Cook the farro with the salt until tender, according to the package directions.

3. Toast the nuts on a rimmed baking sheet in the oven. Shake them after 5 minutes, check after another 3 minutes, and take them out when they look golden and smell nutty, usually after no more than 12 minutes total. Remove from the pan to cool, then chop roughly.

4. Meanwhile, release the pomegranate seeds (see Tip); set them aside.

5. Mix 1 teaspoon of honey into the yogurt in a small bowl.

6. Whisk the vinegar with the remaining 2 tablespoons of honey and the cinnamon in a large bowl. Toss this mixture with the cooked farro.

7. Let it cool to about room temperature, then toss gently with the pomegranate seeds, nuts, and chocolate. Spoon into wine glasses or small mason jars, and top with the sweetened yogurt.

INGREDIENT TIP: To seed the pomegranate without a mess, score it into quarters longitudinally, submerge it in a bowl of water, and pull apart the pieces. Then, use your hands to gently bend the rind backward and coax the seeds out, all under the water. The pith will float, and the seeds will sink. Separate, drain, and enjoy!

PER SERVING: Calories: 274; Total Fat: 12g; Saturated Fat: 3g; Cholesterol: 3mg; Sodium: 61mg; Carbohydrates: 36g; Fiber: 6g; Added Sugars: 11g; Protein: 8g; Potassium: 347mg; Vitamin K: 9mcg

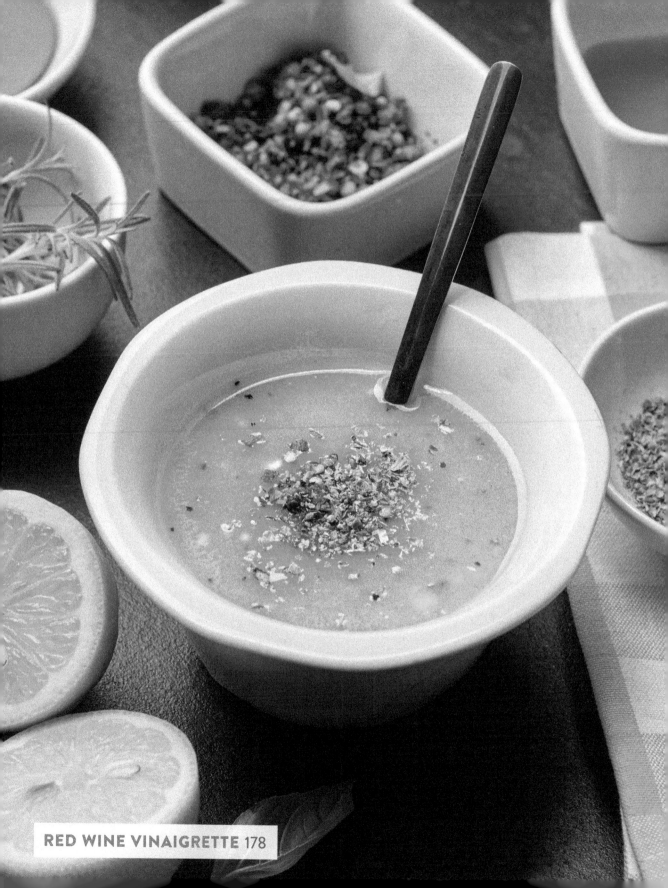

RED WINE VINAIGRETTE 178

CHAPTER NINE

STAPLES

FRUIT-INFUSED SPARKLING WATER

VEGAN • 5-INGREDIENT • NO-COOK • PORTABLE

If water tastes boring but you're trying to avoid juice and other sugary beverages, get creative with naturally flavored sparkling water. There's no limit to the flavors you can add. Try lime with cherries (fresh or frozen), blackberries and fresh mint, pomegranate and cucumber, or strawberries and fresh basil. Crush the fruit if you want the juices to infuse your water faster. This works well with frozen fruit, too. Microwave frozen fruit for a few seconds if you want to drink your infused water right away, or use the fruit straight from the freezer and let the flavor infuse over time.

Serves 2

Hands-on time: 5 min

Total time: 5 min

1 (32-ounce/1 liter) bottle low-sodium club soda or sparkling water

3 orange segments, halved

5 raspberries, halved

1. In a pitcher, combine the club soda and fruit.

2. Drink right away, or prepare in advance for more intense flavor.

COOKING TIP: A lesson I learned the hard way: If you're using a SodaStream to make sparkling water, add any fruit *after* you carbonate the water.

PER SERVING: Calories: 6; Total Fat: 0g; Saturated Fat: 0g; Cholesterol: 0mg; Sodium: 38mg; Carbohydrates: 1g; Fiber: 0g; Added Sugars: 0g; Protein: 0g; Potassium: 18mg; Vitamin K: 0mcg

SALT-FREE SOUTHWEST SEASONING MIX

VEGAN • NO-COOK • PORTABLE

Spices and herbs are the best ways to heighten the flavor of food when you want to cut back on salt. Rather than pull out five or six jars each time you cook, spend a few minutes mixing your favorites. This combination works with a variety of dishes, and you can add or subtract ingredients to taste. Once you've nailed down your favorite combination, double the recipe and you'll be covered for months.

Makes ¼ cup (1 teaspoon per serving)

Hands-on time: 5 min

Total time: 5 min

2 tablespoons chili powder

2 teaspoons garlic powder

2 teaspoons onion powder

1 teaspoon chipotle powder

1 teaspoon dried oregano

1 teaspoon dried thyme

1. Mix the chili powder, garlic powder, onion powder, chipotle powder, oregano, and thyme together in a small bowl.

2. Store in an airtight container.

INGREDIENT TIP: Chipotle powder is made of crushed dried, smoked jalapeño peppers. It imparts a distinctive hot and smoky taste, so increase the amount if you like that or skip it if you don't. Dried herbs and ground spices lose their punch after two to three years. Note the date with a Sharpie when you buy them, and toss any that look, smell, or taste like they're past their prime.

PER SERVING: Calories: 11; Total Fat: 0g; Saturated Fat: 0g; Cholesterol: 0mg; Sodium: 1mg; Carbohydrates: 3g; Fiber: 0g; Added Sugars: 0g; Protein: 0g; Potassium: 13mg; Vitamin K: 2mcg

BETTER BUTTER

VEGETARIAN • 5-INGREDIENT • NO-COOK

This recipe gives you spreadable buttery taste with more heart-healthy unsaturated fats. It's like homemade soft margarine. Use it for spreading on toast, topping steamed vegetables, and anything else you use butter for. Olive oil isn't an ideal choice for this, unless you don't mind the green tint.

Makes about 2 cups
(1 tablespoon per
serving)

Hands-on time: 5 min

Total time: 5 min

1 cup unsalted butter,
softened to room
temperature

1¼ cups canola or
sunflower oil

1. Blend the butter and oil together in the food processor until the mixture is perfectly smooth. It may take 2 to 3 minutes.

2. Pour the mixture into a storage container with a lid. Store in the refrigerator.

COOKING TIP: If you haven't had a chance to soften the butter, purée it first with the food processor, then let it sit for 15 to 20 minutes before proceeding with the recipe.

PER SERVING: Calories: 121; Total Fat: 14g; Saturated Fat: 4g; Cholesterol: 14mg; Sodium: 1mg; Carbohydrates: 0g; Fiber: 0g; Added Sugars: 0g; Protein: 0g; Potassium: 2mg; Vitamin K: 6mcg

LEMON-TAHINI DRESSING

MEDITERRANEAN • VEGAN • NO-COOK • PORTABLE

This dressing is perfect for making a vegetarian or chicken bowl like the Lemon-Tahini and Tofu Energy Bowl (page 96). Improvise a quick meal by drizzling it over Crispy Tofu (page 186) or Pan-Seared Chicken (page 120), raw or steamed vegetables, and a cooked whole grain like quinoa or barley. Use a colorful mixture of vegetables chopped, spiralized, grated, or even sliced paper-thin with a vegetable peeler.

Makes ¾ cup
(2 tablespoons per serving)

Hands-on time: 5 min

Total time: 5 min

⅓ cup extra-virgin olive oil

2 tablespoons nutritional yeast

2 tablespoons freshly squeezed lemon juice

2 tablespoons water

1 tablespoon reduced-sodium tamari

1 tablespoon tahini

1 small garlic clove, minced

1. Mix the olive oil, nutritional yeast, lemon juice, water, tamari, tahini, and garlic in a mini–food processor, or whisk the ingredients by hand in a large bowl.

2. Store in an airtight container in the refrigerator for up to 1 week.

PER SERVING: Calories: 132; Total Fat: 14g; Saturated Fat: 2g; Cholesterol: 0mg; Sodium: 122mg; Carbohydrates: 2g; Fiber: 0g; Added Sugars: 0g; Protein: 1g; Potassium: 42mg; Vitamin K: 7mcg

RED WINE VINAIGRETTE

Although it uses a little salt to heighten the flavor, this simple homemade dressing still has about half the sodium of commercial dressings. Olive oil gets thick and lumpy when refrigerated, but a few minutes at room temperature and a good shake will fix that. Use half a garlic clove in place of the shallot if you like that sharp, raw garlic zing, but it will get more pungent with time. Use garlic powder for a more subtle flavor.

Makes 1 cup
(2 tablespoons per serving)

Hands-on time: 5 min

Total time: 5 min

½ cup extra-virgin olive oil

3 tablespoons red wine vinegar

2 tablespoons Dijon mustard

2 teaspoons honey

1 small shallot, minced (optional)

¼ teaspoon salt (optional)

¼ teaspoon freshly ground black pepper

1. Combine the olive oil, vinegar, mustard, honey, shallot and salt (if using), and pepper in a mini-food processor, or whisk the ingredients by hand in a large bowl.

2. Store in an airtight container in the refrigerator for up to 1 week.

SUBSTITUTION TIP: Substitute maple syrup for the honey for a vegan dressing.

PER SERVING: Calories: 142; Total Fat: 15g; Saturated Fat: 2g; Cholesterol: 0mg; Sodium: 153mg; Carbohydrates: 2g; Fiber: 0g; Added Sugars: 2g; Protein: 0g; Potassium: 13mg; Vitamin K: 9mcg

TOMATO-BALSAMIC VINAIGRETTE

DASH • MEDITERRANEAN • VEGAN • NO-COOK • PORTABLE

This quick vinaigrette makes a flavorful topping for grilled fish, chicken, or meat, thanks to the umami flavor of the balsamic vinegar and tomatoes. In winter, when tomatoes aren't in season, use a handful of chopped cherry or grape tomatoes. Fresh thyme or basil will take this to the next level.

Makes 1 cup (¼ cup per serving)

Hands-on time: 5 min

Total time: 5 min

1 medium ripe tomato, seeded and diced

½ shallot, minced

¼ cup extra-virgin olive oil

2 tablespoons balsamic vinegar

¼ teaspoon freshly ground black pepper

⅛ teaspoon salt

1. Gently mix the tomato, shallot, olive oil. vinegar, pepper, and salt in a large bowl.

2. Store in an airtight container in the refrigerator for up to 1 week.

INGREDIENT TIP: Shallots are a milder tasting onion, so they're good for salad dressing. Yellow onion and garlic are substitutes with stronger flavor, so use just a little if you opt for those. Garlic powder can stand in if you prefer a milder flavor.

PER SERVING: Calories: 133; Total Fat: 14g; Saturated Fat: 2g; Cholesterol: 0mg; Sodium: 76mg; Carbohydrates: 3g; Fiber: 0g; Added Sugars: 0g; Protein: 0g; Potassium: 85mg; Vitamin K: 11mcg

CHIMICHURRI

MEDITERRANEAN • VEGAN • NO-COOK • PORTABLE

Chimichurri is a flavorful fresh herb mixture that originated in Argentina. It's traditionally used with grilled meat, but it makes a delicious topping for chicken and fish, too, as in the Pan-Seared Halibut with Chimichurri Sauce (page 105).

Serves 4

Hands-on time: 10 min

Total time: 10 min

¼ cup extra virgin olive oil

2 tablespoons red wine vinegar

2 shallots, peeled

2 garlic cloves, peeled

¼ cup fresh flat-leaf parsley

¼ cup fresh cilantro

1 teaspoon dried oregano

¼ teaspoon kosher salt

Freshly ground black pepper

1. Combine the olive oil, vinegar, shallots, garlic, parsley, cilantro, oregano, salt, and pepper in a food processor or mini-chopper. Pulse until the herbs are minced but not puréed. If you don't have a food processor, finely chop the shallots, herbs, and garlic, and mix with the other ingredients in a medium bowl.

2. Store in an airtight container in the refrigerator for up to 1 week.

FLAVOR BOOST: Add a finely chopped fresh red chile or a sprinkle of red pepper flakes for more heat.

PER SERVING: Calories: 131; Total Fat: 14g; Saturated Fat: 2g; Cholesterol: 0mg; Sodium: 125mg; Carbohydrates: 2g; Fiber: 1g; Added Sugars: 0g; Protein: 0g; Potassium: 63mg; Vitamin K: 74mcg

WALNUT PESTO

DASH • MEDITERRANEAN • VEGETARIAN • PORTABLE

Pesto is tasty and heart-healthy, but store-bought jars are loaded with salt. Making it yourself means more flavor and antioxidants from basil, extra-virgin olive oil, and nuts. I use walnuts instead of pine nuts because they're less expensive and rich in omega-3 fat. (Although the fat in pine nuts is heart-healthy, too—you can't go wrong!) This has less olive oil and Parmesan than some recipes. If you're using it with pasta, save ½ cup of your pasta cooking water and add that with the pesto. If you're using it on fish or chicken, add a little more olive oil as needed.

Serves 4 (just under ¼ cup per serving)

Hands-on time: 15 min

Total time: 15 min

2 tablespoons walnuts

2 cups loosely packed fresh basil leaves

¼ cup extra-virgin olive oil

1 garlic clove, peeled

⅛ teaspoon salt

⅓ cup grated Parmesan cheese

1. Preheat the oven to 350°F.

2. Toast the nuts on a rimmed baking sheet in the oven. Shake them after 5 minutes, check after another 3 minutes, and take them out when they look golden and smell nutty, usually no more than 12 minutes total. Remove from the pan to cool.

3. Blend the toasted nuts with the basil, olive oil, garlic, salt, and cheese in a food processor.

4. Store in an airtight container in the refrigerator for up to 1 week.

FLAVOR BOOST: Taste, then add another clove or two of garlic, if you like. Substitute arugula for the basil if you like the peppery taste, or try a handful of oil-packed sun-dried tomatoes.

LEFTOVERS: If you're planning to freeze this, leave the cheese out and freeze it flat, with no air bubbles, in a zip-top bag. Break off a piece when needed, and add the cheese just before serving.

PER SERVING: Calories: 173; Total Fat: 18g; Saturated Fat: 3g; Cholesterol: 4mg; Sodium: 164mg; Carbohydrates: 1g; Fiber: 0g; Added Sugars: 0g; Protein: 3g; Potassium: 61mg; Vitamin K: 58mcg

FRESH TOMATO SALSA

DASH • MEDITERRANEAN • VEGAN • NO-COOK • PORTABLE

This quick homemade salsa is bursting with fresh flavor, even though it has just a fraction of the sodium of commercial products. Enjoy it with Baked Tortilla Chips (page 155), over fish or chicken, or with burritos, quesadillas, or tacos. Make things easy by pulsing everything in the food processor rather than chopping by hand.

Serves 8 (¼ cup per serving)

Hands-on time: 15 min

Total time: 15 min

2 cups chopped fresh tomatoes

½ cup chopped fresh cilantro

¼ cup minced red onion

1 medium jalapeño pepper, seeded and minced

3 tablespoons freshly squeezed lime or lemon juice

1 garlic clove, minced

½ teaspoon ground cumin

¼ teaspoon freshly ground black pepper

¼ to ½ teaspoon kosher salt

Mix the tomatoes, cilantro, onion, jalapeño, lime juice, garlic, cumin, pepper, and salt together in a pretty bowl.

INGREDIENT TIP: Add an extra jalapeño if you like more heat. The seeds and ribs are the spiciest part. Include them if you like, but be careful! Wear a pair of clean kitchen gloves, and avoid touching your eyes when cutting any chiles.

PER SERVING: Calories: 13; Total Fat: 0g; Saturated Fat: 0g; Cholesterol: 0mg; Sodium: 123mg; Carbohydrates: 3g; Fiber: 1g; Added Sugars: 0g; Protein: 1g; Potassium: 133mg; Vitamin K: 7mcg

PINEAPPLE-CRANBERRY SALSA

DASH • MEDITERRANEAN • VEGAN • NO-COOK • PORTABLE

Here's a fresh, light, pretty topping for grilled fish, chicken, or pork. It's perfect with summer tacos, too. Add a minced jalapeño or red pepper flakes for more heat. If you can make this an hour or so ahead of time, the flavors will come together beautifully, although it's also delicious eaten right away.

Makes about 1½ cups
(¼ cup per serving)

Hands-on time: 15 min

Total time: 15 min

1½ cups finely diced fresh
pineapple

¼ cup finely chopped
red onion

¼ cup diced bell pepper
(any color)

1 teaspoon minced
fresh ginger

¼ cup chopped fresh
cilantro

1 tablespoon red
wine vinegar

¼ cup dried cranberries

Toss the pineapple, onion, bell pepper, ginger, cilantro, vinegar, and cranberries together in a medium bowl.

COOKING TIP: You can also use canned pineapple chunks in juice, but skip the dried cranberries; it'll be sweet enough.

PER SERVING: Calories: 43; Total Fat: 0g; Saturated Fat: 0g; Cholesterol: 0mg; Sodium: 2mg; Carbohydrates: 11g; Fiber: 1g; Added Sugars: 4g; Protein: 0g; Potassium: 74mg; Vitamin K: 1mcg

BLUEBERRY-CHIA JAM

DASH • MEDITERRANEAN • VEGETARIAN • 5-INGREDIENT • ONE POT • PORTABLE

Traditionally, jam is made with cooked fruit, pectin, and sugar. A lot of sugar. Thickening it with chia seeds instead adds cholesterol-lowering soluble fiber and healthy fats. Fresh fruit works in this recipe, too, but frozen is easier and usually more affordable. Once you see how easy and delicious this is, try it with strawberries, raspberries, blackberries, cherries, or peaches. Use the jam for topping porridge, pancakes, plain Greek yogurt, or peanut butter and toast. For a thicker jam, double the amount of chia seeds.

Serves 4 (¼ cup per serving)

Hands-on time: 5 min

Total time: 15 min

2 cups frozen blueberries

1 tablespoon chia seeds

1 teaspoon honey (optional)

1. Warm the blueberries in a small saucepan over medium heat, stirring occasionally, for about 10 minutes.

2. Once the berries are defrosted and bubbling, remove the pan from the heat and add the honey (if using) and chia seeds.

3. Let it sit at least 5 minutes to thicken.

4. Let the jam cool to room temperature, then store it in an airtight container in the refrigerator for up to 1 week.

INGREDIENT TIP: White chia seeds are preferable if you use a lighter-colored fruit like peaches and don't want to see them. For the blueberries, both white and black chia seeds work just fine.

COOKING TIP: Heat the berries for 1 to 2 minutes in the microwave, then add the honey and chia seeds.

PER SERVING: Calories: 58; Total Fat: 1g; Saturated Fat: 0g; Cholesterol: 0mg; Sodium: 1mg; Carbohydrates: 12g; Fiber: 3g; Added Sugars: 1g; Protein: 1g; Potassium: 53mg; Vitamin K: 13mcg

MUSHROOM AND THYME GRAVY

DASH • VEGETARIAN • ONE POT

Gravy made thick and rich with mushrooms is proof that vegetables don't have to be boring. Cremini and white button mushrooms both work for this, but if you include a portobello or shiitake, you'll get an even deeper, richer flavor. Need more salt? Try a few drops of reduced-sodium tamari or soy sauce—more savory for less sodium.

Serves 4

Hands-on time: 10 min

Total time: 30 min

1 tablespoon Better Butter (page 176) *or* 1½ teaspoons unsalted butter plus 1½ teaspoons extra-virgin olive oil

½ onion, finely chopped

2 garlic cloves, minced

8 ounces sliced mushrooms

¼ teaspoon salt

¼ teaspoon freshly ground black pepper

2 tablespoons all-purpose flour

1 cup reduced-sodium beef broth

1 tablespoon chopped fresh thyme

1 tablespoon half-and-half (optional)

1. Heat the Better Butter in a large skillet over medium heat. When it starts to froth, add the onion, garlic, mushrooms, salt, and pepper. Turn the heat up to medium-high, and cook the mushrooms until browned, about 10 minutes.

2. Stir in the flour and cook, stirring frequently, for about 5 minutes.

3. Add the broth slowly, stirring briskly to incorporate. When it starts to boil, turn the heat down to medium-low. Add the thyme. Simmer for another 10 minutes or so, adding more broth if it gets too thick. Stir in the half-and-half (if using). Taste, and adjust the seasonings.

SUBSTITUTION TIP: Substitute reduced-sodium chicken broth if that's what you have. Substitute a teaspoon of dried thyme if you don't have fresh, or a tablespoon of fresh rosemary.

PER SERVING: Calories: 72; Total Fat: 4g; Saturated Fat: 1g; Cholesterol: 5mg; Sodium: 247mg; Carbohydrates: 7g; Fiber: 1g; Added Sugars: 0g; Protein: 3g; Potassium: 232mg; Vitamin K: 2mcg

CRISPY TOFU

DASH • MEDITERRANEAN • VEGAN • ONE POT • PORTABLE

If you're not a tofu lover, this might convert you. You can skip the garlic, ginger, and tamari sauce if you're using it with Lemon-Tahini Dressing (page 177) or another flavorful sauce. Skip the cornstarch if you're in a hurry—it just won't be as crispy. Stir-in garlic and ginger paste make this a cinch. They're both salted, so cut the tamari in half if you use them.

Serves 4

Hands-on time: 20 min

Total time: 25 min

1 pound extra-firm tofu

¼ cup cornstarch

1 tablespoon canola or sunflower oil

1 garlic clove, minced (optional)

1 teaspoon minced fresh ginger (optional)

2 teaspoons reduced-sodium tamari (optional)

1. Drain the tofu, and slice through its equator to make two flat blocks. Wrap them side by side in a couple of layers of clean kitchen or paper towels, and put a heavy book or frying pan on top for at least 5 minutes.

2. Cut the tofu slabs into 1-inch squares. Put the tofu squares in a zip-top bag or food storage container, and add the cornstarch. Seal the bag and gently turn to coat the tofu pieces on all sides.

3. Heat the oil in a nonstick skillet over medium-high heat. When it is shimmering, add the tofu. Let it cook undisturbed until golden brown on the bottom, about 5 minutes. Flip each piece and cook until crispy on the other side, 4 to 5 minutes more.

4. Add the garlic and/or ginger (if using), and gently stir with the tofu for about 1 minute.

5. Transfer the tofu to a paper towel to soak up any extra oil. Sprinkle with the tamari (if using).

COOKING TIP: A cast iron skillet will give you crispier tofu, but you'll need to double the oil.

PER SERVING: Calories: 160; Total Fat: 8g; Saturated Fat: 1g; Cholesterol: 0mg; Sodium: 123mg; Carbohydrates: 10g; Fiber: 1g; Added Sugars: 0g; Protein: 11g; Potassium: 5mg; Vitamin K: 4mcg

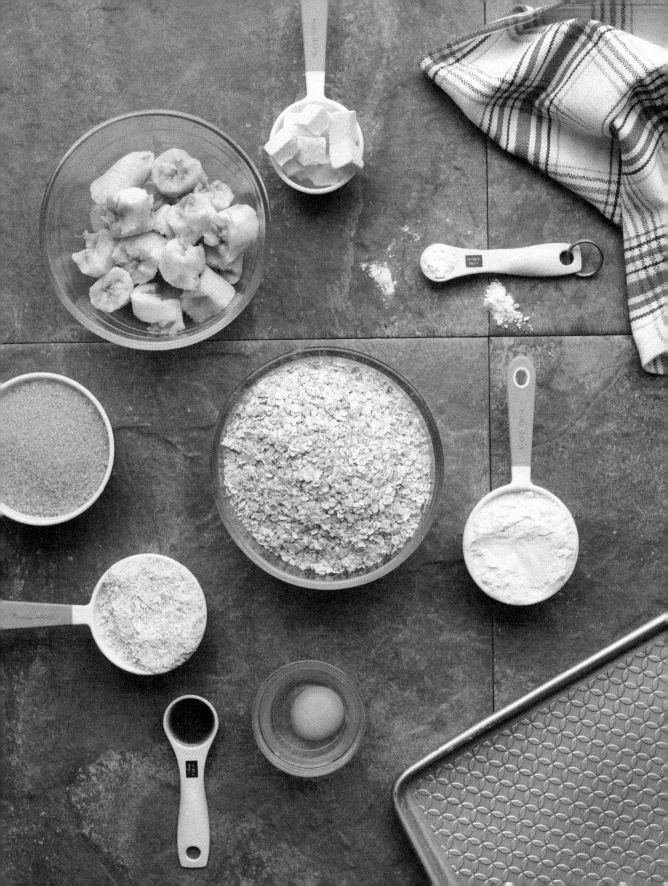

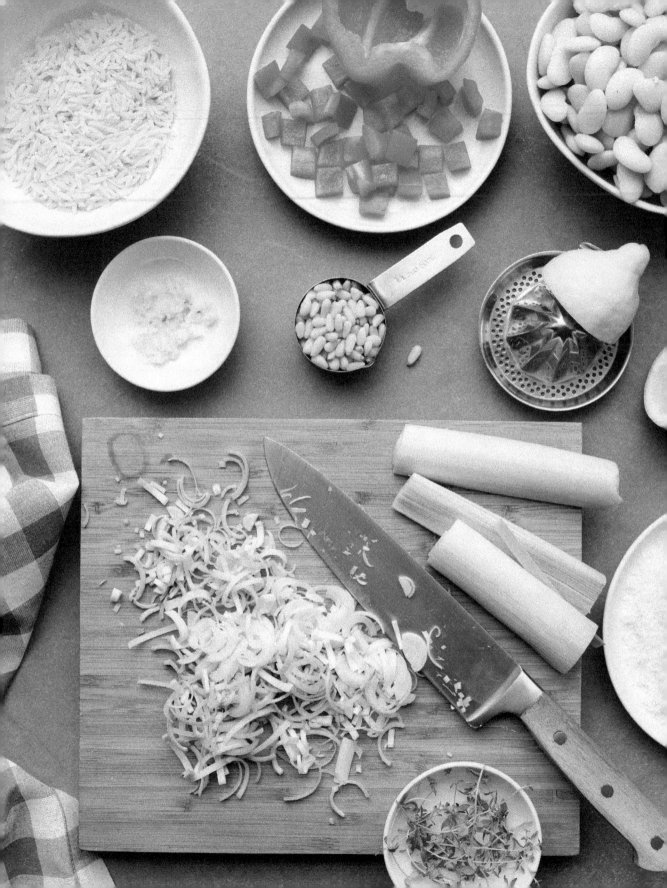

Measurements and Conversions

	US STANDARD	US STANDARD (OUNCES)	METRIC (APPROXIMATE)
VOLUME EQUIVALENTS (LIQUID)	2 tablespoons	1 fl. oz.	30 mL
	¼ cup	2 fl. oz.	60 mL
	½ cup	4 fl. oz.	120 mL
	1 cup	8 fl. oz.	240 mL
	1½ cups	12 fl. oz.	355 mL
	2 cups or 1 pint	16 fl. oz.	475 mL
	4 cups or 1 quart	32 fl. oz.	1 L
	1 gallon	128 fl. oz.	4 L
VOLUME EQUIVALENTS (DRY)	⅛ teaspoon	————	0.5 mL
	¼ teaspoon	————	1 mL
	½ teaspoon	————	2 mL
	¾ teaspoon	————	4 mL
	1 teaspoon	————	5 mL
	1 tablespoon	————	15 mL
	¼ cup	————	59 mL
	⅓ cup	————	79 mL
	½ cup	————	118 mL
	⅔ cup	————	156 mL
	¾ cup	————	177 mL
	1 cup	————	235 mL
	2 cups or 1 pint	————	475 mL
	3 cups	————	700 mL
	4 cups or 1 quart	————	1 L
	½ gallon	————	2 L
	1 gallon	————	4 L
WEIGHT EQUIVALENTS	½ ounce	————	15 g
	1 ounce	————	30 g
	2 ounces	————	60 g
	4 ounces	————	115 g
	8 ounces	————	225 g
	12 ounces	————	340 g
	16 ounces or 1 pound	————	455 g

	FAHRENHEIT (F)	CELSIUS (C) (APPROXIMATE)
OVEN TEMPERATURES	250°F	120°F
	300°F	150°C
	325°F	180°C
	375°F	190°C
	400°F	200°C
	425°F	220°C
	450°F	230°C

References

Advisory Committee, US Department of Agriculture, Agricultural Research Service, "Advisory Report to the Secretary of Health and Human Services and the Secretary of Agriculture." (Washington, 2015). https://health.gov/dietaryguidelines/2015-scientific-report/PDFs/Scientific-Report-of-the-2015-Dietary-Guidelines-Advisory-Committee.pdf.

Anderson, T. J., J. Grégoire, G. J. Pearson, et al. 2016. "Canadian Cardiovascular Society Guidelines for the Management of Dyslipidemia for the Prevention of Cardiovascular Disease in the Adult." *Canadian Journal of Cardiology* 3,2 no. 11 (November 2016): 1263–1282. doi:10.1016/j.cjca.2016.07.510.

Appel, L. J., T. J. Moore, E. Obarzanek, et al. "A Clinical Trial of the Effects of Dietary Patterns on Blood Pressure." *New England Journal of Medicine* 336 (April 1997): 1117–1124 doi:10.1056/NEJM199704173361601.

Appel, L. J., F. M. Sacks, V. J. Carey, et al. "Effects of Protein, Monounsaturated Fat, and Carbohydrate Intake on Blood Pressure and Serum Lipids: Results of the OmniHeart Randomized Trial" *JAMA* 294, no. 19 (November 2005): 2455–2464. doi:10.1001/jama.294.19.2455.

Australian Government, National Health and Medical Research Council, "Clinical Practice Guidelines for the Management of Overweight and Obesity in Adults, Adolescents, and Children in Australia" (Melbourne, 2013). https://www.nhmrc.gov.au/about-us/publications/clinical-practice-guidelines-management-overweight-and-obesity.

Bacon, L., and L. Aphramor. "Weight Science: Evaluating the Evidence for a Paradigm Shift." *Nutrition Journal* 10, no. 9 (January 2011). doi:10.1186/1475-2891-10-9.

Berger, S., G. Raman, R. Vishwanathan, et al. "Dietary Cholesterol and Cardiovascular Disease: A Systematic Review and Meta-Analysis." *American Journal of Clinical Nutrition* 102, no. 2 (June 2015): 276–294. doi:10.3945/ajcn.114.100305.

Chiavaroli, L., S. K. Nishi, T. A. Khan, et al. "Portfolio Dietary Pattern and Cardiovascular Disease: A Systematic Review and Meta-analysis of Controlled Trials." *Progress in Cardiovascular Diseases* 61, no. 1 (May 2018): 43–53. doi:10.1016/j.pcad.2018.05.004.

Chiu, S., N. Bergeron, P. T. Williams, G. A. Bray, et al. "Comparison of the DASH (Dietary Approaches to Stop Hypertension) Diet and a Higher-Fat DASH Diet on Blood Pressure and Lipids and Lipoproteins: A Randomized Controlled Trial." *American Journal of Clinical Nutrition* 103, no. 2 (February 2016): 341–347. doi:10.3945/ajcn.115.123281.

Collins, K. "The Debate about Dietary Cholesterol: Should Nutrition Recommendations Set a Limit?" American College of Cardiology (August 2015). https://www.acc.org/latest-in-cardiology/articles/2015/08/19/12/57/the-debate-about-dietary-cholesterol.

de Lorgeril, M., P. Salen, J. Martin, et al. "Mediterranean Diet, Traditional Risk Factors, and the Rate of Cardiovascular Complications after Myocardial Infarction." *Circulation* 99, no. 6 (February 1999): 779–785. doi:10.1161/01.CIR.99.6.779.

Dietary Guidelines Advisory Committee, Office of Disease Prevention and Health Promotion. "Scientific Report of the 2015 Dietary Guidelines." https://health.gov/dietaryguidelines/2015-scientific-report/.

Huang, T., B. Yang, J. Zheng, et al. "Cardiovascular Disease Mortality and Cancer Incidence in Vegetarians: A Meta-Analysis and Systematic Review." *Annals of Nutrition & Metabolism* 60, no. 4 (June 2012): 233–240. doi:10.1159/000337301.

Iestra, J., K. Knoops, D. Kromhout, et al. "Lifestyle, Mediterranean Diet and Survival in European Post-Myocardial Infarction Patients." *European Journal of Cardiovascular Prevention and Rehabilitation* 13, no. 6 (December 2006): 894–900. doi:10.1097/01.hjr.0000201517.36214.ba.

Li, S., S. E. Chiuve, A. Flint, et al. "Better Diet Quality and Decreased Mortality Among Myocardial Infarction Survivors." *JAMA Internal Medicine* 173, no. 19 (October 2013): 1808–1819. doi:10.1001/jamainternmed.2013.9768.

Mann, T. A., J. Tomiyama, E. Westling, et al. "Medicare's Search for Effective Obesity Treatments." *American Psychologist* 62, no. 3 (April 2007): 220–233. doi:10.1037/0003-066X.62.3.220.

Marcus, J. B. "Smoke Points of Common Fats and Oils." In *Culinary Nutrition: The Science and Practice of Healthy Cooking* (Cambridge, Mass.: Academic Press, 2013).

Miller, M., N. J. Stone, C. Ballantyne, et al. "Triglycerides and Cardiovascular Disease." *Circulation* 123, no. 20 (May 2011): 2292–2333. doi:10.1161/CIR.0b013e3182160726.

Mozaffarian, D. "Dietary and Policy Priorities for Cardiovascular Disease, Diabetes, and Obesity: A Comprehensive Review." *Circulation* 133, no. 2 (January 2016): 187–225. doi:10.1161/CIRCULATIONAHA.115.018585.

NIH Technology Assessment Conference Panel. "Methods for Voluntary Weight Loss and Control." *Annals of Internal Medicine* 116, no. 11 (June 1992): 942–949. doi: 10.7326/0003-4819-116-11-942.

Ornish, D., S. E. Brown, J. H. Billings, et al. "Can Lifestyle Changes Reverse Coronary Heart Disease? The Lifestyle Heart Trial." *Lancet* 336. no. 8708 (July 1990): 129–133. doi:10.1016/0140-6736(90)91656-U.

Sacks, F. M., A. H. Lichtenstein, J. H. Y. Wu, et al. "Dietary Fats and Cardiovascular Disease: A Presidential Advisory From the American Heart Association." *Circulation* 136, no. 3 (July 2017): e1–e23. doi:10.1161/CIR.0000000000000510.

Salehi-Abargouei, A., Z. Maghsoudi, F. Shirani, et al. "Effects of Dietary Approaches to Stop Hypertension (DASH)-Style Diet on Fatal or Nonfatal Cardiovascular Diseases—Incidence: A Systematic Review and Meta-Analysis on Observational Prospective Studies." *Nutrition* 29, no. 4 (2013): 611–618. doi:10.1016/j.nut.2012.12.018.

Sievenpiper, J. L., C. B. Chan, P. D. Dworatzek, et al. "Diabetes Canada 2018 Clinical Practice Guidelines for the Prevention and Management of Diabetes in Canada: Nutrition Therapy." *Canadian Journal of Diabetes* 42 (2018): S88–S103. https://guidelines.diabetes.ca/cpg/chapter11.

Sotos-Prieto, M., S. N. Bhupathiraju, J. Mattei, et al. "Association of Changes in Diet Quality with Total and Cause-Specific Mortality." *New England Journal of Medicine* 377 (July 2017): 143–153. doi:10.1056/NEJMoa1613502.

Spaeth, A. M., D. F. Dinges, and N. Goel. "Effects of Experimental Sleep Restriction on Weight Gain, Caloric Intake, and Meal Timing in Healthy Adults." *Sleep* 36, no. 7 (July 2013): 981–990. doi:10.5665/sleep.2792.

Tokede, O. A., T. A. Onabanjo, A. Yansane, et al. "Soya Products and Serum Lipids: A Meta-Analysis of Randomised Controlled Rrials." *British Journal of Nutrition* 114, no. 6 (September 2015): 831–843. doi:10.1017/S0007114515002603.

Tribole, E., and E. Resch. *Intuitive Eating: A Revolutionary Program that Works* (New York: St. Martin's Griffin, 2012).

Tylka, T. L., R. A. Annunziato, D. Burgard, et al., "The Weight-Inclusive versus Weight-Normative Approach to Health: Evaluating the Evidence for Prioritizing Well-Being over Weight Loss." *Journal of Obesity* (July 2014). doi:10.1155/2014/983495.

Van Horn, L., J. S. Carson, L. J. Appel, et al. "Recommended Dietary Pattern to Achieve Adherence to the American Heart Association/American College of Cardiology (AHA/ACC) Guidelines." *Circulation* 134, no. 22 (November 2016): e505–e529. doi:10.1161/CIR.0000000000000462.

Index

ACKNOWLEDGMENTS

I'm incredibly grateful to the community of people who helped bring this book to life, from dietitian Kristyn Hall, with her culinary expertise and friendship, to other dietitians who jumped in at a moment's notice to test, measure, and help perfect recipes: Vincci Tsui, Carolina Leon, Jayne Thirsk, Karyn Sunohara, Melissa Conniff, Marni Larsen, Linda Cuda, Renee Little, Andrea Clarke, Grace Wong, Sarah Kish Higgins, Julia MacLaren, Piper Quickstad, and dietetic intern Britney Lentz.

Thanks to my sister Tracy Kelly and cousin Tara Sawatzky for their meat-cooking savvy, as well as the friends who paused their busy lives to try recipes and offer valuable feedback: Heidi Phan-Peterson, Laura Mytels, Denise Yamamoto, Michele Peart, Lorraine Rawson, Stacey Squires, and Alissa Nicolucci.

Thanks to the many food writers, instructors, and passionate cooks who've taught and inspired me, particularly Calgary's Julie Van Rosendaal.

Finally, thanks to Callisto Media editor Clara Song Lee for recognizing the need for heart-healthy food that can fit into people's real lives, and trusting me to write this, as well as editor Beth Adelman, for her expertise, flexibility, and patience.

ABOUT THE AUTHOR

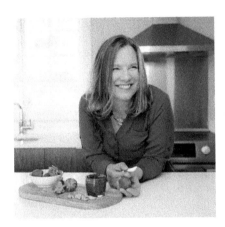

CHERYL STRACHAN is a registered dietitian, speaker, and writer who specializes in cardiac health and is on a mission to help people with heart concerns relax about food and enjoy cooking, eating, health, and happiness.

She has provided nutrition counseling and education to thousands of people, between the TotalCardiology Rehabilitation program and her private practice, Sweet Spot Nutrition, in Calgary, Canada. You can follow her mostly weekly blog for cardiac nutrition demystification, inspiration, and perspective at sweetspotnutrition.ca.

When she's not tinkering in the kitchen, writing, or making unrealistically long to-do lists, Cheryl plays basement volleyball with her two tireless daughters, walks a small dog with a big bark, and counts the hours until date night with her sweet husband.